Flexible Dieting IIFYM

Featuring Flexible Dietin Cookbook

Copyright © 2014 by Scott James

All rights reserved.

Contents

Calories:

Disclaimer

The information provided in this book is designed to provide helpful information on the subjects discussed. This book is not meant to be used, nor should it be used, to diagnose or treat any medical condition. For diagnosis or treatment of any medical problem, consult your own physician. The publisher and author are not responsible for any specific health or allergy needs that may require medical supervision and are not liable for any damages or negative consequences from any treatment, action, application or preparation, to any person reading or following the information in this book. References are provided for informational purposes only and do not constitute endorsement of any websites or other sources. Readers should be aware that the websites listed in this book may change.

I recommend consulting a doctor to assess and/or identify any health related issues prior to making any dramatic changes to your diet.

About the Author

Scott James has been addicted to all things fitness, health and nutrition for nearly a decade.

With a large amount of hype surrounding the fitness industry, as well as the dieting and supplementation niches Scott thought it was the right time to come forward and debunk the myths and scams within the industry.

All information conveyed in Scott's books is tried and tested - no false hope or bad information is shared.

Scott believes that when an individual is equipped with the correct knowledge and a plan of action that he will provide in his books they are unstoppable.

Scott is not here to make money, he's here to make a different and guide you on your journey to unlocking the new, better you.

Bonus Content

As a token of my appreciation, I'd like to give you access to my exclusive bonus content.

Here's what you're about to receive...

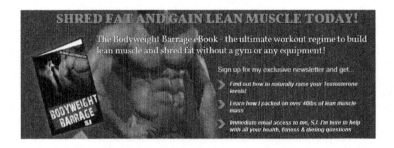

- **The Bodyweight Barrage eBook - the ultimate guide to building muscle and shredding fat without a gym, including exercise descriptions, photos and more!**

- **Immediate email access to me, SJ. Ask me anything, and I'll give you an answer**

- **My honest product reviews and recommendations**

In order to claim your bonus content, simply navigate to:

http://ignorelimits.com/bwbarrage

Enter your email in the box so you can receive this exclusive content instantly!

As this is a limited time offer I recommend claiming your Bodyweight Barrage ebook before proceeding to read the book.

Introduction – A Paradigm Shift

First of all, I'd like to say thank you for purchasing this e-book! You've just taken the first step in turning the body of your dreams into a reality.

You are reading this book because an element of your current diet is insufficient – it could be due to minimal or no results, or because you are not enthusiastic about the limited range of foods your current 'diet' allows you to eat. Food is essentially fuel for the body, and I will show you how to fuel your body with the foods of your choice. Low carbohydrate diets often leave you feeling sluggish and result in poor performance in sports and day to day activities– this book does not preach low carbohydrates or 'crash' diets.

After years of reading and applying knowledge of dieting from various sources and seeing amazing results using a flexible dieting approach, I thought there should be a simple easy to follow guide documenting the new craze that is flexible dieting. Unfortunately, the only books available seem to contain questionable information and lots of 'filler' material; needless to say, I began work on creating a book that contains the truth.

All of the information contained within this guide is tried and tested – so all you have to do is follow the information I am about to present to you. There is no guess work involved - all you have to do is take action!

How many times have you been told that certain foods, such as ice cream, chocolate or anything particularly high in carbohydrates, will make you fat? Or that steamed vegetables and boiled chicken is the diet you must endure in order to achieve the body of your dreams? That has been the train of thought for the last few decades, but no more. Flexible dieting (also known as IIFYM 'if it fits your macros') is the way to live a balanced lifestyle while still creating and maintaining the physique of your dreams.

I will teach you why starving yourself and 'crash diets' actually hinder your weight loss progress, and how to go about fixing this as well as the most effective ways to measure your progress (instead of stepping on the scale).

<u>The clean eating myth has been debunked.</u>

The human body is a regulated system, it does not want to lose fat or gain muscle. Just like the cruise control in your car or heating/cooling system in your house, the human body regulates a variety of elements (such as your body temperature and metabolism) to maintain its current state. After reading this book, you will be equipped with the knowledge to outsmart the body and efficiently achieve the physique of your dreams!

I hope you enjoy reading this book as much as I enjoyed writing it.

What is Clean Eating?

Clean eating (also known as the 'bro' diet) until recently has been believed as the only way to lose fat and build a 'fitness model' or 'bikini' style physique.

For a food to be known as 'clean,' it must contain no preservatives, refined sugars, trans fats or have undergone any processing – essentially if it didn't exist 100 years ago or cannot be found around the perimeter of your local grocery store (fresh produce, meat, seafood and dairy), it does not fit into the category of clean food. Diets that are comprised of these clean foods are simply plain and dull, lacking flavour and variety due to the fact that so few foods meet this criterion.

A typical clean eating diet will contain:

Protein sources such as

- Boiled Chicken
- Kangaroo Steaks
- Lean Steak
- Turkey
- Grilled Fish
- Egg Whites

Carbohydrate sources such as

- Wholemeal Bread
- Brown Rice
- Oatmeal
- Sweet Potato

- Steamed Vegetables
- Fresh Fruit

Fat sources such as

- Almonds
- Organic Peanut Butter
- Tuna
- Olive Oil
- Eggs (whole)

A clean eating diet comprised of the foods listed above is realistically very hard to sustain; a newcomer will be enthusiastic for several days, a week or perhaps even a month - but over time the strict discipline required to adhere to this form of diet will more often than not turn them off dieting and lead them to consider weight loss to be near impossible. This is where flexible dieting comes to the rescue!

What is Flexible Dieting (IIFYM)?

Flexible dieting is more of a lifestyle then an actual diet. Flexible dieting eliminates 'clean' and 'dirty' foods and instead focuses on the bigger picture – your daily caloric needs (which I will show you how to calculate later in this book). Flexible dieting thrives on the principle that a calorie is a calorie and which source it comes from will have no effect on body composition. You can gain fat eating 'clean' foods if you exceed the daily amount of calories your body requires, just like you can lose fat eating 'dirty' foods as long as the total calories consumed are below that of your maintenance level.

Post-workout is the ideal time to consume carbohydrates to restore your glycogen levels and to replenish the muscles after they have been torn to shreds (the process of receiving a 'pump' when lifting weights is the process of healthy ripping and bleeding of muscle fibres). Flexible dieting means that 50 grams of carbohydrates consumed from brown rice will have the same effect on your body as 50g of carbohydrates consumed from Coco Pops.

The clean eating myth has been debunked.

Flexible dieting will allow you to include your favourite foods in your diet, as long as they fit within your calorie goal. Some of the foods I consume on a regularly basis as part of my diet include:

- Smoothies
- Poptarts
- Cheesecake

- Pizza
- Subway
- Hamburgers

Benefits of Flexible Dieting (IIFYM)

Flexibility

I bet you can now see why Flexible Dieting has quickly become a new craze, as it is just that – flexible. No longer do you have to worry about which foods you can and can't eat, so long as they meet your caloric requirements – you are not limited to a minute range of food.

Minimal impact on social life

How many times have you been invited out to a meal or social event with friends, but have had to decline due to your 'clean diet?' With flexible dieting, this is no longer the case; you don't make friends with salad.

Sustainability

Flexible dieting is sustainable - you can eat foods you enjoy daily and will, therefore, not get cravings to binge on a huge amount of 'junk' food as you would if you were following a 'clean eating' diet. This is often the breaking point for many newcomers to the world of fat loss and dieting.

Preparation Time

With flexible dieting comes a lot of spare time! Following a strict clean eating diet that contains no processed foods means a lot of time is spent cooking, steaming and generally preparing your daily meals. Flexible dieting is fast and efficient, as minimal preparation is required – you can easily hit your caloric goal for the day with takeaway food while out and about if need be.

No Further Eating Disorders

Clean eating encourages disordered eating behaviour which, in turn, creates unnecessary stress. With IIFYM, you will no longer feel guilty as you are no longer chained to a small list of 'allowed' foods. If you have been preaching clean eating for a prolonged period of time, this paradigm shift may take some time.

Results

IIFYM works. By calculating your required daily caloric intake and macronutrient breakdown you will get results. Don't believe me?

Professor Mark Haub – This Kansas State nutritionist experimented with flexible dieting in 2010 in order to prove to his students that 'clean eating' was not the only way to lose fat. During Mark's experiment he lost a massive 27lbs over the course of 10 weeks, and this phenomenon was blogged about all over the internet as 'Professor loses 27lbs on Twinkie diet.' Mark's diet consisted 80% of food purchased through convenience stores, with the remaining 20% of his intake coming from vegetables, protein shakes and a multivitamin (1800 calories per day). This is not classified as a rapid 'crash' diet as Mark's maintenance calories would have been around 2300~ calories, a 500 calorie deficit as recommended to strip fat.

Mark not only lost 27lbs but his health indicators also improved – HDL and LDL cholesterol as well as triglyceride. Mark's justification for this experiment was to demonstrate to students that "in weight loss pure calorie counting is what matters most, not the nutritional value of the food."

Cardio

So, to get the body of your dreams, do you need to partake in hours of mind numbing cardio such as walking on the treadmill or stair climbing?

The answer to the above question is: certainly not.

The primary purpose of aerobic exercise is to increase the heart rate in order to burn more calories. If excess calories are not consumed, then cardio is not required, it really is that simple – many professional bodybuilders are so precise with their caloric intake that they are able to obtain a competition level physique (3-4% body fat with masses of lean muscle) just through diet manipulation alone!

If you do, however, surpass your caloric target for the day, then cardio can be a very handy tool to offset these excess calories. But don't forget "you can't out train a bad diet." If you calculate your calories using this method, I will present to you further in this book that you will not be required to do any cardio.

> I personally incorporate small amounts of cardio (in the form of high intensity intervals) into my routine to lose the last few pounds of fat instead of dropping my calories lower once I have recalculated my TDEE. TDEE and calculations will be discussed a bit later on in this book.

Note: aerobic activities are fantastic for cardiovascular health, increasing performance in sports, speed and agility, etc. However, that is outside the scope of this book.

Calories

So what is a calorie?

A calorie is an energy source. Humans require calories in order to maintain life. We are constantly trying to increase and decrease our caloric intake based on our goals, such as: whether we want to slim down, gain lean muscle mass or perform a certain way for sports. If a calorie that is consumed is not utilised, it will be converted by the body and stored as fat.

Calories can come from several different macronutrient sources. These include:

Protein – 4 calories per gram– protein serves as building blocks for lean muscle mass.

Carbohydrates – 4 calories per gram – carbohydrates are used by our bodies as the primary energy source. Carbohydrates are broken down into 2 sub categories (both contain 4 cal/gram).

Simple carbohydrates – these are the sugary processed carbohydrates that are found in foods such as lollies, chocolate and fruit. Simple carbohydrates are absorbed quickly and cause a large insulin spike.

Complex carbohydrates – These carbohydrates are the 'clean' slow digesting carbohydrates that are known for sustained energy. Complex carbs are found in brown rice, sweet potato and oats.

Fat – 9 calories per gram – Healthy fats are vital for bodily functions such as hormone levels. Fats are also broken down into several categories:

Saturated fat – found in dairy and meat, can raise cholesterol.

Unsatured fat – found in vegetable oils, used to lower cholesterol.

Alcohol – 7 calories per gram – empty calories (alcohol does not contain any macronutrients).

Calculating Your Macronutrients

In order to begin your flexible diet, you need to know your daily caloric goal! Be sure to have a calculator or degree in mathematics on hand. In order to calculate this goal, the following formula is used (please note the slight variation in formula for men and women):

Based on the extremely accurate Mifflin - St Jeor equation

MEN: BMR = [9.99 x weight (kg)] + [6.25 x height (cm)] - [4.92 x age (years)] + 5

WOMEN: BMR = [9.99 x weight (kg)] + [6.25 x height (cm)] - [4.92 x age (years)] -161

The above equation will give you your BMR – this is your Basal Metabolic Rate. In other words, the number of calories your body needs to function while at rest.

You then multiply the BMR by an 'activity variable' to obtain your TDEE (total daily energy expenditure). This Activity Factor is the cost of living and it is based on more than just your workouts. It also includes work/lifestyle, sports andand the thermogenic effect of food (essentially the amount of energy burned in the process of digesting food).

 Average activity variables are as follows:

1.2 = Sedentary - Little or no exercise + desk job

1.3-1.4 = Lightly Active - Little daily activity and light exercise 1-3 days a week

1.5-1.6 = Moderately Active - Moderately active daily life and moderate exercise 3-5 days a week

1.7-1.8 = Very Active - Physically demanding lifestyle and hard exercise or sports 6-7 days a week

1.9-2.0 = Extremely Active - Hard daily exercise or sports and physical job

Below are some examples of this calculation performed correctly:

Male

90kg male – 21 years old - 187cm tall – desk job, minimal exercise

[9.99 * 90] + [6.25 * 187] – [4.92 * 21] – 5 * Activity Level 1.2 = 2350 calories

70kg male – 18 years old - 170cm tall – physical job, lots of exercise

[9.99 * 70] + [6.25 * 170] – [4.92 * 18] – 5 * Activity level 1.7 = 2852 calories

Female

65kg female – 28 years old – 140cm – desk job, minimal exercise
[9.99 * 65] + [6.25 * 140] – [4.92 * 28] – 161 * Activity level 1.2 = 1500 calories

55kg female – 18 years old – 150cm – moderately active
[9.99 * 55] + [6.25 * 150] – [4.92 * 18] – 161 * Activity
level 1.5 = 1414 calories

Alternatively, you can use an online calculator based off
the Mifflin – St Jeor equation, please refer to the 'Useful
Links' section at the end of this book.

Goal Based Calorie Consumption

Now that you have calculated your TDEE (Total Daily Energy Expenditure), you need to determine what your goal is. Do you want to maintain your current state? Do you want to strip fat? Do you want to pack on lean muscle?

The biggest mistake being made when deciding to lose weight is to go into a starvation or 'crash' diet. Dropping to 1000~ calories per day will initially give you a period of weight loss at an impressive rate, however, this WILL cause metabolic damage (the process of your body rapidly decreasing it's metabolism and the rate at which calories are burned due to the minimal amount of food it is receiving, essentially going into survival mode). Also, you guessed it: the only way to repair a damaged metabolism is to slowly start to eat more. Crash dieting is not sustainable - do not do it.

For weight loss – consume 500 calories below your TDEE per day.

For lean muscle gain – consume 500 calories above your TDEE per day.

To maintain – consume the exact number of calories as your TDEE each day.

As your progress begins to slow down, it is time to re-calculate your TDEE via the same formula you used previously (listed above) as you will now find that your TDEE has changed! As you add lean mass, your TDEE will considerably increase. As you begin to lose weight, you will notice your TDEE has decreased (and, therefore, after a month you only be eating 200 calories under your TDEE instead of the 500 calories that you were initially consuming under).

Note: I personally recalculate TDEE on a monthly basis; I recommend you do the same.

Calorie Macronutrient Breakdown

Now that we have determined your calorie goal, and established that you can eat which ever foods you choose to reach this magical caloric value, it is important to establish an accurate ratio of protein, carbohydrates and fats to consume.

For optimal performance in sports and resistance training (as well as to keep your appetite in check), I recommend consuming at least 30% of your daily calories from protein, with the remaining 70% coming from a breakdown of calories and fats.

You'll notice in the common macronutrient splits listed below, the percentage of calories derived from fat does not drop below 20%. This is due to the fact that hormones are constructed from cholesterol along with other fat molecules; dropping the percentage of fat consumed any lower can suppress your normal hormone levels. Why is this an issue, you ask? Because these hormones drive the growth and development of your body, your metabolism, reproduction system and mood. Low fat intake causes deficiency in essential fatty acids and also highly increases your risk of cancer.

Although, as stated, you will lose fat simply by consuming under your TDEE calories and gain weight by eating above your TDEE, I would highly recommend following a high protein approach. If you neglect your protein intake, you will not build and retain lean muscle. Meals high in protein will also keep you feeling fuller for longer, unlike those rich in carbohydrates and fats.

Note: When referring to a macronutrient breakdown, the order listed is Protein:Carbohydrates:Fat

Common macronutrient splits include:

30P:50C:20F
moderately high protein, high carbohydrate, low fat. Often used when going through a mass building or 'bulking' phase.

35P:40C:30F
moderately high protein, moderately high carbohydrates, higher fats than usual. This is a reasonably even split of macronutrients, and I would recommend this style of macronutrient split when maintaining your current body composition.

40P:40C:20F
High protein, high carbohydrates, and low fat. The most commonly used macronutrient split used by bodybuilders and fitness enthusiasts today, used for both fat loss and addition of lean muscle mass simply by adjusting the number of calories consumed.

50P:30C:20F
High protein, low carbohydrate, low fat. This macronutrient split is often used for ongoing fat loss diets, as the high protein content keeps the individual feeling quite full and content between their meals. With this low level of carbohydrates, refeeds are necessary (this will be discussed further in the book).

35P:60C:5F
Moderate protein, high fat, minimal carbohydrates. A diet comprised of these macronutrients is known as a

'ketogenic diet.' The primary purpose of this diet is to adjust the body to use fat as the primary stored energy source as opposed to carbohydrates – when the body enters this state (which takes several days) it is in a state of ketosis. I would not recommend following this style of macronutrient breakdown due to the previously mentioned hormone suppression that occurs with low fat diets. Food choice is also extremely limited to essentially meats, nuts and a small portion of vegetables, which defeats the purpose of flexible dieting.

Personal Note:

I follow a 40:35:25 macronutrient breakdown.

For example – I am currently consuming 2800 calories to trim the last bit of body fat; my daily macronutrient breakdown is 280 grams of protein per day, 245 grams of carbohydrates per day and 78 grams of fats per day.

Required Macronutrients

Fiber

Fiber is an essential macronutrient that our body requires for aiding digestion. A 'clean eating' diet comprises of lots of foods that contain high fiber content – however, while flexible dieting, it is equally important that we meet our fiber needs.

Women need to aim for 22 – 28 grams of dietary fiber per day.

Men need to aim for 28 – 34 grams of dietary fiber per day.

There are a range of fiber supplements available on the market, however, these are (as the name suggests) only a supplement to your regular fiber intake. Foods high in fiber include whole grains, fruits and vegetables (note: these are all forms of carbohydrates).

Refeeds

What is a Refeed?

If you are embarking on a fat loss journey through the use of flexible dieting (or any style of dieting!) it is paramount to incorporate structured refeeds. Please note that this section is irrelevant if you intend to follow a calorie surplus to gain lean mass. A structured refeed is a 24 hour period in which you drastically alter your macronutrient breakdown after being in a calorie deficit (consuming fewer calories than your TDEE).

Why is a Refeed Essential?

A refeed will boost your metabolism and assist in restoring your Leptin hormone levels - Leptin is the king of all fat burning hormones. When in a calorie deficit, your metabolism will drop (meaning less calories are being burnt), plus your leptin hormone levels will drop in attempt by the body to spare body fat. This is a safety mechanism put in place for the body.

We need to understand that our body is resistant to change, no matter what our current body composition is - our body does not want to change. The human body does not want to lose fat; it simply wants to survive. Consuming below your TDEE (Total Daily Energy Expenditure) will force your body to slow down your metabolism, resulting in a lower caloric intake to continually burn body fat.

As the metabolism begins to slow and Leptin levels drop, it becomes a lot harder to burn excess body fat.

26

Therefore, including a refeed day into your diet will encourage your body to burn fat at a consistent rate.

The leaner you are, the more often you will need to refeed; lower body fat = lower leptin levels. This is based upon body fat percentage; you will learn how to calculate this in the section below.

Refeed Frequency

Body fat Percentage	Frequency of Refeed
Over 20%	Monthly
15 – 20%	Fortnightly
10 – 15%	Weekly
Under 10%	Twice Weekly

Please refer to the following table for refeed timing:

Carbohydrate Intake During a Refeed

On your structured refeed day, I recommend you leave your protein and fat intakes the same as any other day. However, double your carbohydrate intake for this 24 hour period. This will put you slightly over your maintenance calories for the day, but it will have long term benefits (as discussed above).

Here is an example of my regular caloric intake:

2800 calories (500 below my TDEE)
280 grams of protein
245 grams of carbohydrates
78 grams of fats

Here is my typical caloric intake on a structured refeed day:

3780 calories (580 calories above my TDEE)
280 grams of protein
490 grams of carbohydrates
78 grams of fats

As we have previously addressed, a carbohydrate is a carbohydrate – you can derive these extra carbohydrates from whichever source you choose, it does not matter whether they are simple or complex. On a refeed day, I typically indulge in oats, ice cream, pancakes, bananas and pasta as these are all very rich in carbohydrates.

Flexible Dieting Recipes

The next 3 pages contain a few of my favourite flexible dieting meals. These are easy to fit into your daily macronutrients and very easy to make. I am far from a master chef, so if I can make these - so can you. I eat these meals on a regular basis.

If you enjoy these recipes, be sure to stay tuned for a dedicated recipe and protein smoothie book which I will be releasing in the near future.

Protein Power Pizza

Description:

A succulent miniature protein pizza, this recipe can be altered to suit your personal preference, however, this is a great base to work with.

Ingredients:

Wholemeal Pita Bread
Tomato Paste
Whole Chicken
Baby Spinach
Tomatoes
Mushroom
Cheese (if desired)

Method:

- Spread tomato paste over wholemeal pita bread base
- Cut up chicken and place on pizza (1 whole chicken = 6 pizzas)
- Cover pizza with spinach, mushroom and tomato
- Place pizzas in over on 200 degrees Celsius (392F) for 20 minutes

Macronutrients

Per pizza

Protein: 50g
Carbohydrates: 45G
Fat: 5G

425 calories

Premium Protein Cheesecake

Description:

Delicious protein cheesecake, this cheesecake can be made in different variations simply by altering the flavour of protein used (change vanilla to chocolate and add some topping) or stick with vanilla and add some berries.

Ingredients:

340 grams (12oz) fat free cream cheese
280 grams (10oz) plain greek yoghurt
2 eggs
2 tbsp stevia
¼ cup of milk
2 scoops whey protein
1 tsp vanilla extract
Dash of salt

Method:

- Preheat oven to 160 degrees Celsius (320F)
- Soften cream cheese in a large mixing bowl
- Add eggs and stevia, proceed to mix
- Add the remaining ingredients
- Mix all ingredients for 3 minutes
- Pour mixture into baking pan lined with parchment paper
- Bake at 160 degrees Celius (320F) for 20 minutes then adjust to 90 degrees Celsius (194F) for an hour
- Place in fridge for 5 hours to cool
- Serve with toppings if desired

Macronutrients
per 225 grams (8oz) slice

40g protein
15g carbohydrates
2g fat

238 calories

Mad Monkey Protein Smoothie

Description:

A thick and delicious chocolate smoothie that packs a punch! Great for increasing your energy level before a workout.

Ingredients:

2 scoops chocolate whey protein
100ml skim milk
1 banana
1 tblspn peanut butter
1 tspn coffee
1 cup ice

Method:

- Place all ingredients in a blender or magic bullet and blend for ~20 seconds
- Enjoy!

-
-
-

- **Macronutrients:**

55g protein
32g carbohydrates
15g fat

401 calories

Meal Timing

I'm sure you've heard this before: in order to achieve your fitness goals, you need to eat a larger number of smaller meals (for example 5 – 6 meals a day). This, along with clean eating, is preached heavily by nutritionists and personal trainers.

What if I told you meal frequency and nutrient timing doesn't matter at all? Or that eating 6 times a day will have no effect on your metabolism or metabolic rate? That you can eat carbs right before bed and you won't gain fat?

Upon first thinking about this, it may sound like I'm making this all up. Surely consuming food prior to sleeping will be stored as fat as you are not actively exercising to utilise these calories. However, our body does not operate like this – it is constantly looking at the bigger picture, the calories/macronutrients we consume over a 24 or 48 hour period. Your body is constantly breaking down and repairing itself, storing and oxidizing nutrients.

It's hard to instantly change your beliefs on an aspect of fitness that is constantly preached, but a paradigm shift is required – individuals spend far too much time stressing over the timing of their meals and how many they consume a day rather than focusing on the most important aspect of dieting.

<u>Eat what you want, when you want - as long as you hit your caloric goal.</u>

A study on the "Effect of the Pattern of Food Intake on Human Energy Metabolism" states:

The pattern of food intake can affect the regulation of body weight and lipogenesis. We studied the effect of meal frequency on human energy expenditure (EE) and its components. During 1 week ten male adults (age 25-61 years, body mass index 20.7-30.4 kg/m2) were fed to energy balance at two meals/d (gorging pattern) and during another week at seven meals/d (nibbling pattern). For the first 6 d of each week the food was provided at home, followed by a 36 h stay in a respiration chamber. O2 consumption and CO2 production (and hence EE) were calculated over 24 h. EE in free-living conditions was measured over the 2 weeks with doubly-labelled water (average daily metabolic rate, ADMR). The three major components of ADMR are basal metabolic rate (BMR), diet-induced thermogenesis (DIT) and EE for physical activity (ACT). There was no significant effect of meal frequency on 24 h EE or ADMR. Furthermore, BMR and ACT did not differ between the two patterns. DIT was significantly elevated in the gorging pattern, but this effect was neutralized by correction for the relevant time interval. With the method used for determination of DIT no significant effect of meal frequency on the contribution of DIT to ADMR could be demonstrated.'

Please refer to Appendix A for the details of 3 other case studies on nutrient timing to solidify the fact that meal timing is indeed irrelevant for body composition.

One factor to take into account regarding meal timing is your energy levels. Some individuals yield better results in terms of energy when consuming a meal an hour before a workout, others prefer to train fasted. This comes down to personal preference and, as I have stressed, will have no effect whatsoever on overall body composition.

Before we delve deeper into the following sections, it is imperative we clarify weight loss and fat loss.

Weight loss is one of the most lucrative topics in existence. The majority of people claim that they want to lose weight or fat, interchangeably switching between both of these hot keywords – little do they know there is a big difference between the two.

Weight Loss refers to your complete body weight; this is the sum of your bones, muscles, organs, water and fat.

Fat Loss refers to the amount of fat you are carrying on your body, measured as a percentage of your total body weight.

When weight loss is discussed, I'm sure you can now see that this is indeed a reference for people wanting to lose fat. In the 'tracking progress' section below, I will show you how to accurately assess your fat loss progress if this is indeed your goal.

The major issue when discussing 'weight loss' is how unreliable it is. Your total weight fluctuates daily based upon stomach, bowel and bladder content, water loss and retention; with a large carbohydrate intake, water is bound (this is why a low/no carb diet will initially give you an impressive decrease in weight, as you no longer retain anywhere near as much water). Muscle loss and gain as well as fat loss and gain also play a major role. Researchers refer to those who lose weight easily but find it harder to gain weight to be 'spendthrift' with those that are able to gain weight easily but have more of an issue losing weight to be 'thrifty' – this ties in with the body types listed below.

There are 3 classic 'body types' in existence, some individuals are a mix of more than 1 of these, however, it is very important to know which category you fall under as this can play a large role on your style of training and caloric intake – for example, an ectomorph (often referred to as skinny) has a harder time gaining weight then the other 2 body types and will, therefore, need to slightly up their caloric intake – although they do not need to drop their calories very low to promote fat loss.

Below are diagrams and common traits of each of the 3 body types – which one are you?

Ectomorph

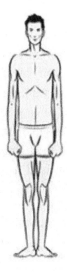

- Skinny slender frame
- Small joints
- Long limbs
- Narrow shoulders
- Fast metabolism
- Hard to gain weight
- Easy to lose weight

Endomorph

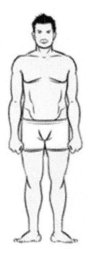

- Soft, chubby frame
- Puts on both weight and muscle with ease
- Finds weight loss hard
- Short and stocky
- Minimal muscle defintiion
- Slow metabolism

Mesomorph

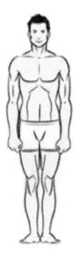

- Naturally athletic
- Define muscles 'hard' looking body
- Strong
- Gains muscle easy
- Gains fat easier than an ectomorph

Now that you have determined your body type based off the above common traits, you can fine tune your workout routine and caloric intake to suit it.

Personal Note: I am an Ectomorph, also known as a 'hard gainer,' therefore, in order for me to put on lean mass, I have to consume a slightly larger number of calories due to a fast metabolism (600 calories over my TDEE as opposed to the standard 500). While trying to add lean mass, I avoid large amounts of cardio as ectomorphs lose weight easily, which is counterproductive to my goals.

Trial and error is the only way to find what will produce the best results for you.

"In order to know where we're going we must first know where we are and where we have been." – Greg Plitt

When you get in your car, you have an end destination in mind, along with check points on the way to this destination. In your weight loss/mass gain diet, these progress checks are your check points, while your dream body is the destination.

Tracking progress is essential, without regularly checking your progress you won't know whether your current training regime and caloric intake are suitable for you.

Most individuals simply rely on the scales to track progress; don't fall into the trap of weighing yourself daily. Remember: weight constantly fluctuates based on the time of the day as well as other factors, such as fluid intake, meals consumed, stress and a number of other factors. Therefore, I personally deem the methods below, along with a weigh in on the scales once a week (first thing in the morning prior to consuming any food), to be the most accurate way to determine whether you're making progress.

Realistic expectations - I am not here to tell you that you're going to lose 20kg of fat in 5 weeks, or that you can stack on lean muscle in a few days of hitting your caloric goal. These results are simply not attainable. Consistent results are the best kind of results. Following a ketogenic or low carbohydrate diet will initially give you a large period of weight loss as this is the process of your body losing water weight due to a decrease in carbohydrates (as water binds to carbohydrates). But, soon after that the progress will diminish. Please refer to the following figures which are ideal for consistent fat loss.

Body Composition	Estimated Consistent Loss
Lean (<15%)	1lb per week
Average (15 – 20%)	2lbs per week
Overweight (>20%)	4lbs per week

Measurements

Use a tape measure and measure the circumference of your neck, chest, biceps, waist, thighs and calves. Record these measurements in a Microsoft Excel spread sheet weekly. Here is an example:

Body Part	Week 1	Week 2	Week 3
Neck (circumference, cm)	42cm	41cm	40.5cm
Chest	68cm	68cm	69cm
Biceps (average of 2)	35cm	35cm	36cm
Waist	80cm	79cm	77cm
Thighs (average of 2)	60cm	59cm	58.5cm
Calves (average of 2)	40cm	40cm	40cm

Based on the example table above, you can see that the sizes of this individuals arms and chest are increasing, while their waist and thighs have slowly started to decrease. Tracking progress via these measurements allows us to see which body parts are progressing and which are lagging behind – adjustments to your routine can then be made to counteract this.

Photos

Take photos of your physique on a weekly basis, including front, side and rear views of your physique. When taking these progress photos, ensure they are taken in the same location at the same time of day consistently (I would recommend first thing in the morning) to avoid any differences in lighting and water retention from food, etc. This is to ensure you capture the most accurate representation of your physique each time – making it easy to gauge progress. Print out these photos and stick them on your bathroom mirror; record your weight and body measurements on the back. There is no better motivation then seeing your hard work transform into progress.

Body Fat Percentage

If you have access to a body fat caliper, it is recommended you also measure your body fat percentage every 2 weeks. Body fat calipers can be purchased online for as little as $4 and come with full instructions on how to accurately measure your body fat. The most common and accurate sites to measure from include your pectoral, triceps, lats, lower abdomen and thigh.

Others methods used to measure your body fat percentage include:

Body fat scales - An electric current are pulsed through your body and uses biometrical impedance analysis to analyze the amount of body fat you are holding. I would not recommend using this method as

the result given can vary dramatically based on the amount of water you are holding.

The measurement method - By taking measurements using the US Navy body fat calculating technique, you can calculate your body fat percentage. A link to calculate your body fat using this method is located in the 'Useful Links' section at the end of this book.

DEXA Scanning- Dexa scanning is undoubtedly the most accurate method as it takes a full X-ray of your body composition and gives you the numbers. Dexa scans are performed at specialized health clinics; the process of getting a Dexa scan involves you lying on an X-Ray table for 15 minutes. It's typically very expensive, coming in at around the $200 mark, although, as stated, it is the most accurate method.

Looking
If you are familiar with what a male or female body looks like at certain body fat levels, you can simply gauge where you are currently in comparison. A chart below showing both male and female physiques at different body fat percentages will assist you if this is the method you choose to use.

This, however, is not the method I recommend for measuring ongoing progress (as if you lose 1% body fat over the course of a week or two, it can be hard to distinguish from simply looking). That is where a caliper is best used.

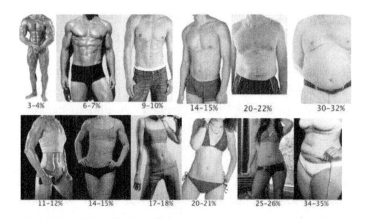

| 3-4% | 6-7% | 9-10% | 14-15% | 20-22% | 30-32% |

| 11-12% | 14-15% | 17-18% | 20-21% | 25-26% | 34-35% |

Clothing

That favourite shirt of yours that you want to fill out or those jeans you haven't been able to comfortably fit in for the last couple of years are a great way to gauge your progress. Over time, you will start to see the composition of your body change. If you're adding lean mass, you will notice your shirts start to fit tighter around the arms. Your shoulder will fill out the shirt more as your waist begins to decrease in circumference.

BMI

BMI, short for body mass index, is a standard measurement used to determine whether an individual is within the 'healthy' weight range for their height.

A person's BMI is calculated as their weight in kilograms divided by their height in meters, squared. A BMI of 18.5

to 24.9 is considered within the 'normal' range, a BMI between 25 to 29.9 is said to be 'overweight,' and a BMI greater than 30 is classed as 'obese.' The majority of studies done relating to overweight individuals reference their BMI. I do not recommend anybody use BMI as a measure of progress or to determine whether they are 'in shape.'

BMI is completely flawed. BMI only takes into account the height and weight of an individual; it does not take into account many other important factors, such as muscle mass, bone density, body composition, racial and sex differences.

For example, a muscular individual 6'1 weighing 250lbs with a body fat percentage of 8% will have the same BMI result as a 200lbs 6'1 individual weighing 200lbs with 30% body fat.

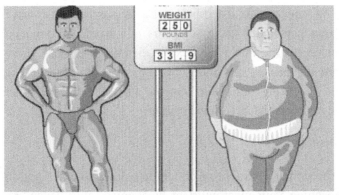

The image above sums up the issue with BMI. Both of these individuals are deemed 'obese' according to the healthy range of BMI results.

Fitness supplements are a multi-billion dollar industry – but do all the supplements on the market do what they claim? Certainly not. No powder will 'Increase your bench press by 128% as proven by college studies' or give you the 'ripped abs you deserve, in 3 weeks or less.' If it sounds too good to be true, it probably is. Supplements serve the purpose they suggest: they simply 'supplement' your diet. Providing you are hitting your caloric intake and macronutrients each day, supplementation may contribute up to 5%.

As long as newcomers continue to get conned into purchasing all of these magical powders and pills, the supplementation industry will continue to thrive. Did you know that many supplements don't even undergo any testing or approval before they are allowed to be sold on the shelves?

The supplements listed below are the supplements I have been personally using for years and would recommend incorporating into your flexible dieting meal plan. These are the basics, and they have been proven true, unlike many of the other supplements full of fluff and filler ingredients that are on the market.

Protein

The primary purpose of protein powder is to assist you in reaching your macronutrient breakdown, and, depending on your daily intake, it can be hard (and time consuming) to get your protein intake for the day in via solid food –

this is where protein powder comes in to play. 1 scoop of protein powder has between 25 and 30 grams of protein.

Protein is protein. It doesn't vary as much between brands as the manufacturers will lead you to believe. No protein is twice as effective as another, so why should you pay twice as much? Keep it simple and get the right type of protein as opposed to focusing on the brand.

WPI (Whey Protein Isolate)
Whey Protein Isolate is a fast acting type of protein. It begins working almost immediately and is best suited to a post-workout meal. It has no other place in your diet.

WPC (Whey Protein Concentrate)
This is a much cheaper version of WPI, and acts over a much longer period of time. This can be used at any time, but still doesn't compare to, for example, egg protein, as far as effectiveness. WPC is a lot cheaper than WPI and is almost as good; it really provides value for the money.

Casein Protein (Slow Release)
This is a slow acting protein, and generally lasts about 5 hours in your system. This is ideal before bed, or for a midnight snack. If you have the budget, I'd purchase some of this just to take before bed as it will fuel your body for quite some time.

Multivitamin

Multivitamins can greatly help your diet. They're ideal for helping to supplement the vitamins and minerals that your body is deficient in. Some of these you could possibly miss by having a flexible diet. When putting together a diet, we quite often limit how much variety we have. This will lead to us neglecting vital vitamins. The best way to take care of this is simply taking a decent multivitamin. Most of them on the market are fairly priced and provide you with everything you will need from vitamin B to Zinc.

Fish Oil

Fish oil contains EFA (essential fatty acids). It is available in both capsule and liquid form and has many benefits, including a healthier blood cholesterol profile and improved bone health – no more squeaky joints! It also assists in protecting against major diseases, such as cancer. Fish oil also assists in increasing the serotonin levels within your body which results in an overall increase in happiness and well-being. Recent studies also show that fish oil may have an influence on muscle protein synthesis.

When selecting fish oil, ensure it is high in EPA/DHA as these are the main omega 3 fatty acids.

I recommend consuming between 2 – 3G per day (capsules generally come in 1000mg and 1500mg).

Vitamin C

No other vitamin has as many positive effects on the body as vitamin C. As vitamin C is not stored in your body, it needs to be replenished daily. Without supplementation, reaching your daily vitamin C intake can be quite difficult.

Vitamin C is required for the growth and repair of tissues in all parts of your body. It is used to form collagen, a protein used to make skin, scar tissue, tendons, ligaments, and blood vessels. It is also essential for the healing of wounds, and for the repair and maintenance of your cartilage, bones, and teeth. Vitamin C also helps with blood pressure by strengthening the walls of your arteries. It can also prevent damage to cells caused by aging as well as help reduce levels of stress.

For athletes, vitamin C will keep testosterone levels high by supporting a lower ratio of cortisol to testosterone. This will help your body keep up that top level of performance you require on a daily basis.

I recommend consuming 1g of vitamin C per day. As vitamin C is water soluble, any excess amount of this vitamin will simply be urinated out within 24 hours.

> Note: If you begin to feel like you are developing a cold, increase your dosage of vitamin C by 200 – 300 % (often referred to as megadosing).

Caffeine/Coffee

Caffeine is an alkaloid compound found in the seeds, leaves and fruits of various plants. Caffeine is a mild stimulant and drug that acts upon the brain and central nervous system. According to The New York Times, caffeine is known as "the most popular drug used in sports today." Caffeine is apparent in coffee, tea, and pre-workout supplements and capsules to name a few variations.

Caffeine has been involved with many studies over the years, reinforcing its positive effects in fat loss, mental focus and overall physical performance.

The greatest benefit of having caffeine before your workout is its fat burning properties. High amounts of caffeine in black coffee will increase your metabolism, which makes you burn more calories throughout the day. Having coffee before exercise enhances that effect. Also, caffeine and other compounds found in coffee act as an appetite suppressant, making you consume less overall.

Several studies have demonstrated a link between caffeine intake before exercise and increased athletic performance. A report published in *Sports Medicine* refers to caffeine as a "powerful ergogenic aid," and mentions that athletes can "train at a greater power output and train longer" after caffeine consumption. Another study published in the *British Journal of Sports Science* found that subjects who consumed coffee before running 1500 meters on the treadmill completed their run 4.2 seconds faster than the control group, on average. To gain an extra edge in your training sessions, coffee might be just what you need.

Along with increased energy to push through tough workouts, caffeine provides an increase in mental focus as well. Improved focus will help keep workouts productive and effective.

Researchers at the University of Illinois found that subjects who consumed caffeine prior to exercise experienced less muscle pain during their workout than their non-caffeinated counterparts. What conclusion can we draw from this? You can complete more reps at a higher resistance during your weight training sessions, and run faster and longer during your cardio workouts with the assistance of caffeine.

Consuming caffeine in the form of coffee helps protect your body from diseases. Coffee contains large amounts of antioxidants, which protect against damage from free radicals. According to a 2011 study published in *Critical Reviews in Food Science and Nutrition*, coffee consumption has an inverse correlation with diabetes, Parkinson's disease, Alzheimer's disease, and certain forms of cancer.

I recommend consuming 200 – 300mg of caffeine before your workouts (in the form of black coffee), however, individuals have different stimulant tolerances. I would experiment with various doses, but do not exceed this amount. It is beneficial to 'cycle' caffeine as the human body quickly builds a tolerance to the stimulant properties of caffeine and will, therefore, not be as effective. A 1:1 on:off ratio works well.

Cycling caffeine 101

I personally consume caffeine for 10 consecutive days followed by a 10 day recovery period so I don't build a tolerance to the amount used.

Sustainability of Flexible Dieting

How sustainable is flexible dieting? Can you continuously eat delicious foods of your choice and consistently make progress?

Of course! Flexible dieting/IIFYM will continue to work as long as you are reaching your calorie/macronutrient goal and recalculating your TDEE on a regular basis. However, if you intend to follow a flexible dieting approach for a long period of time, there are a few points that must be addressed

- Constantly deriving your carbohydrates from simple sugars can lead to adverse health conditions, such as increased blood sugar levels (which can lead to diabetes), high blood pressure and more. I regularly have check-ups with my local general practitioner to ensure all my levels are within a healthy, normal range.

- If you are not including a variety of vegetables within your diet, I continue to stress the importance of getting in your daily vitamins and minerals via the supplementation of a multivitamin.

- Ensure you are reaching your fiber intake for the day before you consume all of your carbohydrates.

- You should time your meals based around your workout schedule. You should consume a pre-workout meal 60 – 90 minutes before training, comprised of protein and complex carbohydrates for energy. Immediately after your workout is the ideal time to consume simple carbohydrates (chocolate, lollies, etc.) to refuel your glycogen stores (which are now depleted from stressful exercise). You will not make any additional weight loss/gains by doing this. However, for overall energy and recovery pre- and post-workout nutrition are vital.

- The primary purpose of IIFYM is to achieve your desired body composition. It does not emphasise overall heart or organ health, unlike clean eating. Therefore, from a health perspective, it is worth adapting the theory and principles behind IIFYM into your diet, as opposed to literally eating sugar ridden lollies as your primary source of carbohydrates.

Dieting is something we all talk about. People often search for the perfect diet, following each new fad as it appears, hoping that this will be the one that will allow us to make progress. Unfortunately, there is much more chance of failure with each 'fasting' or 'caveman diet' that we try... not necessarily because they don't work, but because they are not something which we can follow over a prolonged period. Any diet that leaves you feeling deprived is almost certainly bound for failure, as is one that leaves you bored with the foods that you are allowed to eat. The ONLY way to successfully make progress towards your goals is to change the way you eat.

Flexible dieting will allow you to incorporate the foods you love into your diet in moderation and still make weight loss progress (or lean muscle gains, depending on your goal). There will no longer be the need to stress about what you can eat when you go out socially as certain foods are no longer labelled as 'bad' or 'fattening.' Now that you know how to calculate and track your daily intake, you can look forward to your next meal instead of dreading the thought of having to consume tasteless boiled vegetables.

For me personally, flexible dieting is the key to living a balanced healthy lifestyle in a body I am proud to own. Setting goals and achieving them with the help of flexible dieting creates new found confidence in the individual which, in turn, motivates you to stay true to the path of the ongoing journey – it is the flow of positive, constant progression. You're either spiralling up or spiralling up.

I hope you enjoyed reading this book as much as I enjoyed creating it for you. I would like to wish you the best of luck with your flexible dieting, so go out there and achieve your goals!

Alberto Nunez on Flexible Dieting

http://www.youtube.com/watch?v=f99jPRSgVjg

Video clip of Alberto Nunez – 3D Muscle Journey Natural Bodybuilding Coach - discussing flexible dieting and IIFYM.

BMI Calculator

http://www.heartfoundation.org.au/healthy-eating/Pages/bmi-calculator.aspx

As far as the BMI calculator, I do not recommend using it as a measurement of progress as stated. But, it is interesting to see whether you fit within the supposed 'healthy' weight range. If you have any reasonable amount of lean muscle mass, you will be classified as 'overweight.'

Body Fat Measurement

Fitness.Bizcalcs.com/Calculator.asp?=Body-Fat-Navy

Online body fat calculator based on the US Navy's method.
I have personally found this method to be accurate within 1 – 2% of using a calculator.

Calorie Calculator

www.Calculator.net/Calorie-Calculator.html

This website features a calculator based on the Mifflin – St Jeor formula. If you are unable to calculate your daily calorie intake using the formula mentioned, I would recommend using this calculator.

Caloric Information

http://www.calorieking.com/

Great website for referencing calories. This site divulges calories in just about everything – and it also has a logging feature similar to that of MyFitnessPal.

Daily Calorie Logger

www.MyFitnessPal.com

This is your new best friend. Create an account on MyFitnessPal and record your meals daily to ensure you are meeting your caloric goals. MyFitnessPal also has iPhone and Android Apps available so you can log your calories while on the go!

Additional Content from the Author

www.FlexibleDieting101.com/Bonus

As a display of my gratitude for downloading this book I encourage you to visit my website, dedicated to the very topic of flexible dieting.

By subscribing here you will receive additional FREE content on the topic of flexible dieting as well as IIFYM tips, tricks and more information tailored for the truth, to help you achieve your goals.

Aerobic Exercise:

Exercise that increases the need for oxygen.

Anaerobic Exercise:

Exercise that focuses primarily on muscular strength and endurance.

BMI:

Body Mass Index. Measure for human body composition based off the individuals height and weight. It is used universally, but it's known to be completely inaccurate.

BMR:

Your Basal Metabolic Rate is an estimation of the number of calories you burn over a 24 hour period at rest.

Body Composition:

A term used to reference the amount of fat (percentage), bone density and lean muscle mass in the human body.

Caffeine:

An alkaloid compound found in tea and coffee plants, primarily used for stimulation of the central nervous system.

Calorie:

A unit of heat used to indicate the amount of energy that a food will produce in the human body.

Carbohydrate:

An organic compound comprised of carbon, hydrogen and oxygen.
4 calories per gram.

Clean Eating:

Only consuming unprocessed foods low in sugar with no preservatives or additives.

Cortisol:

Hormone found in the human body, released when stressed.

Crash Diet:

A weight loss diet undertaken with the aim of extremely rapid results in a short period, thus requiring an unhealthily large calorie deficit. Unsustainable.

Dexa Scan:

The most accurate means of measuring bone mineral density and body fat percentage.

DHA:

Docosahexaenoic Acid is a long-chain fatty acid – belongs to the OMEGA 3 family.

Dirty Food:

Processed foods, often containing high amounts of sugar, carbohydrates and preservatives.

Ectomorph:

A lean and delicate built body, often referred to as a 'hard gainer.'

Endomorph:

A soft, round body with a large proportion of fat tissue.

EPA:

Eicosapentaenoic Acid is a long-chain fatty acid – belongs to the OMEGA 3 family.

Fat Loss:

The process of losing fat, not to be confused with weight loss.

Fiber:

The part of the plants we eat that we cannot fully digest.

Flexible Dieting:

A style of diet that does not label any foods as 'clean' or 'dirty.'

IIFYM:

'If it Fits Your Macros' is a revolutionary new style of diet that relies of calculating the macronutrient content of foods to meet your daily caloric goal.

Leptin:

A hormone produced by the body to regulate energy intake and expenditure.

Macronutrient:

The three main chemical compounds food in food, protein, carbohydrates and fats.

Mesomorph:

A compact and muscular style physique.

Metabolic Damage:

The process of your metabolism slowing down after a sustained period of being in a large calorie deficit or starvation diet.

Metabolism:

The ongoing chemical process that occurs within our body to maintain life.

Micronutrient:

Nutrients required by humans in small dosages to orchestrate a range of physiological functions.

Protein:

Large biological molecules consisting of one or more chains of amino acids. Protein is required for growth and maintenance of the human body.

Saturated Fat:

Found in animal products and processed foods, such as meats, dairy products, chips, and pastries. The chemical structure of a saturated fat is fully saturated with hydrogen atoms, and does not contain double bonds between carbon atoms.

Simply Carbohydrate:

Sugary carbohydrates that are broken down quickly by our body for use as energy. Made up of just one or two sugar molecules.

Spendthrift

Researchers refer to those who lose weight easily but find it harder to gain weight to be spendthrift.

TDEE

Total Daily Energy Expenditure is the total number of calories your body burns over the course of 24 hours sleeping, working, exercising and digesting food.

Thrifty

Researchers refer to individuals that gain weight easily but have more of an issue losing weight to be thrifty.

Unsaturated Fat:

Unsaturated fat is found in foods such as nuts, avocados, and olives. They are liquid at room temperature and differ from saturated fats in that their chemical structure contains double bonds. Additionally, studies have shown that unsaturated fats are also heart-healthy fats.

Weight Loss:

The process of losing body weight; includes water weight.

Appendix A

Studies on Meal Timing

Effect of the Pattern of Food Intake on Human Energy Metabolism

http://www.ncbi.nlm.nih.gov/pubmed/8399092?ordinalpos
=2&itool=EntrezSystem2.PEntrez.Pubmed.Pubmed_Resul
tsPanel.Pubmed_DefaultReportPanel.Pubmed_RVDocSu
m

This study compared 5 meals a day to 2 meals a day, both with the same total caloric intake. The conclusion of this study came to be: "With the method used for determination of DIT no significant effect of meal frequency on the contribution of DIT to ADMR could be demonstrated."

Meal Frequency and Energy Balance

http://www.ncbi.nlm.nih.gov/pubmed/9155494

This is some-what of an analysis of ALL studies done regarding meal frequency and energy expenditure (calories burnt). It essentially states that most studies are neutral on the matter; it states that meal frequency has no effect on metabolism. The VERY few studies saying otherwise were likely flawed.

Optimal Protein Intake and Meal Frequency to Support Maximal Protein Synthesis and Muscle Mass

http://www.slideshare.net/biolayne/optimal-protein-intake-and-meal-frequency-to-support-maximal-protein-synthesis-and-muscle-mass

That is a slideshow produced by Dr. Layne Norton. It essentially shows that protein synthesis is not related to an absolute increase in plasma amino levels, which would be sustained by frequent meals. It's hypothesized that plasma amino spikes are able to stimulate protein synthesis at a much greater rate. This would actually support eating less frequently rather than more frequently.

Reduce Meal Frequency without Calorie Restriction in Normal Middle Aged Adults

http://www.ncbi.nlm.nih.gov/pubmed/17413096

Here's another study that may be taking this myth and completely reversing it. It demonstrated that although eating one meal/day as opposed to three caused an increase in hunger, it actually caused a decrease in fat mass. It also showed a decrease in the catabolic hormone cortisol.

Appendix B

Studies on Nutrient Timing

Whey and Casein and Muscle Protein Synthesis: Effect of Resistance Exercise and Protein Ingestion

http://www.ncbi.nlm.nih.gov/pubmed/21045172

This study showed that immediate responses to whey and casein ingestion were different, but the end result was the same. They both stimulated protein synthesis equally.

Ingestion of Casein and Whey Proteins Result in Muscle Anabolism after Resistance Exercise

http://www.ncbi.nlm.nih.gov/pubmed/15570142

This study shows almost exactly the same thing. Both proteins caused equal protein synthesis.

These findings are only compounded by having solid pre-workout nutrition. A quote by Alan Aragon states: "Properly done pre-workout nutrition EASILY elevates insulin above and beyond the maximal threshold seen to inhibit muscle protein breakdown. This insulin elevation resulting from the pre-workout meal can persist long after your resistance training bout is done. Therefore, thinking you need to spike anything is only the result of neglecting your preworkout nutrition."

Introduction

Cooking - it's either something you love or something you hate, and funnily enough this perception is more often than not based on your cooking abilities! As a health and fitness advocate I have spent endless hours in the kitchen trying to follow complex recipes with obscure ingredients and utensils I didn't have to create bland meals I didn't enjoy.

If you are on a 'diet' or trying to gain lean muscle you will more than likely have gone through a phase of desensitizing yourself to foods, don't worry I went through that stage too! Cooking is meant to be fun, after several years of trial and error in the kitchen I have compiled 160 of my favorite muscle building and fat burning recipes that are easy to make and don't require any complex ingredients or utensils.

The recipes within this book include breakfasts, main meals, snacks and desserts, protein smoothies and sides. All of these meals are loaded with flavour, and even better they are loaded with protein and nutrients. Every recipe has the total number of calories along with a macronutrient breakdown stating the amount of protein, carbohydrates and fats per serve (measured in grams).

If you're anything like me you'll have a sweet tooth for berry pancakes, Boston cream donuts and a variety of other mouth-watering sweet foods. In this book I will show you how to EASILY make these and be able to incorporate them into your diet DAILY if you wish while still achieving your fat loss/muscle gain goals.

It's time to debunk the 'clean eating' myth!

First of all, let's clarify flexible dieting. Flexible dieting is more of a lifestyle then an actual diet. Flexible dieting eliminates 'clean' and 'dirty' foods and instead focuses on the bigger picture – your daily caloric needs. Flexible dieting thrives off the principle that a calorie is a calorie and which source it comes from will have no effect on body composition. You can gain fat eating 'clean' foods if you exceed the daily amount of calories your body requires just like you can lose fat eating 'dirty' foods as long as the total calories consumed are below that of your maintenance level.

IIFYM, short for 'If it Fits Your Macros' refers to choosing foods that fit your daily macronutrient goal.

This cookbook contains a plethora of delicious recipes, all with macronutrient breakdowns; therefore you know exactly how many grams of protein, carbohydrates and fat are within each recipe along with the total caloric number that you can then use to reach your caloric goal for the day.

So what is a calorie?

A calorie is an energy source, humans require calories in order to maintain life. We are constantly trying to increase and decrease our caloric intake based on our goals such as: whether we want to slim down, gain lean muscle mass or perform a certain way for sports. If a calorie that is consumed is not utilised it will be converted by the body and stored as fat – this calorie could be from a stick of celery or a scoop of ice cream, it is irrelevant.

Calories can come from several different macronutrient sources, these include:

Protein – 4 calories per gram– protein is the building block for lean muscle mass.

Carbohydrates – 4 calories per gram – carbohydrates are used by our bodies as the primary energy source. Carbohydrates are broken down into 2 sub categories (both contain 4 cal/gram).

Simple carbohydrates – these are the sugary processed carbohydrates that are found in foods such as lollies, chocolate and fruit. Simple carbohydrates are absorbed quickly and cause a large insulin spike.

Complex carbohydrates – These carbohydrates are the 'clean' slow digesting carbohydrates that are known for sustained energy. Complex carbs are found in brown rice, sweet potato and oats.

Fat – 9 calories per gram – Healthy fats are vital for bodily functions such as hormone levels. Fats are also broken down into several categories:

Saturated fat – found in dairy and meat, can raise cholesterol.

Unsatured fat – found in vegetable oils, used to lower cholesterol.

Alcohol – 7 calories per gram – empty calories (alcohol does not contain any macronutrients).

Calculating your Macronutrient Requirement

In order to begin your flexible diet you need to know your daily caloric goal! In order to calculate this goal the following formula is used, please note the slight variation in formula for men and women:

Based on the extremely accurate Mifflin - St Jeor equation

MEN: BMR = [9.99 x weight (kg)] + [6.25 x height (cm)] - [4.92 x age (years)] + 5

WOMEN: BMR = [9.99 x weight (kg)] + [6.25 x height (cm)] - [4.92 x age (years)] -161

The above equation will give you your BMR – this is your Basal Metabolic Rate. In other words the number of calories your body needs to function while at rest.

You then multiply the BMR by an 'activity variable' to obtain your TDEE (total daily energy expenditure). This Activity Factor is the cost of living and it is based on more than just your workouts. It also includes work/lifestyle, sport & the thermogenic effect of food, (essentially the amount of energy burned in the process of digesting food).

Average activity variables are as follows:

1.2 = Sedentary - Little or no exercise + desk job

1.3-1.4 = Lightly Active - Little daily activity & light exercise 1-3 days a week

1.5-1.6 = Moderately Active - Moderately active daily life & Moderate exercise 3-5 days a week

1.7-1.8 = Very Active - Physically demanding lifestyle & Hard exercise or sports 6-7 days a week

1.9-2.0 = Extremely Active - Hard daily exercise or sports and physical job

This number you have now calculated is the number of calories you need to consume to maintain your current weight.

If your goal is to lose weight, subtract 500 calories from this number and consume the specified amount of calories on a daily basis.

If your goal is to gain lean mass add 500 calories to this number and consume the specified amount of calories on a daily basis.

For a more in depth explanation of the principles and guidelines of Flexible Dieting and IIFYM consider reading the precursor to this book.

'Flexible Dieting 101: Eat the Foods you Love and Achieve the Body of Your Dreams'

Now that you have obtained your magic caloric number from the formula above let's step into the kitchen and create some great meals to help you reach your caloric goal!

From here on in you will find 160 of my favorite flexible dieting recipes, each recipe is categorized under a heading as to the most appropriate use or time to consume the particular meal.

Each recipe states the number of servings, as well as the calorie and macronutrient breakdown on a per serving basis.

Please note that these macronutrients and calories listed with each recipe are calculated using the exact ingredients in the recipe, If you wish to substitute ingredients bear in mind that this will adjust the macronutrient breakdown and calorie total of that meal.

Protein Pancakes

Oatmeal & Egg Whites

Light Breakfast

Scrambled Eggs with Spelt Flakes

Breakfast Fajitas

Big Breakfast Pizza

Vanilla Protein Porridge

Chocolate Peanut Butter & Banana Oatmeal

Apple Cinnamon Oatmeal

Peanut Butter, Banana Oat Breakfast Cookies

2 Minute Pancakes

French Toast Cups

Mocha Oatmeal

Banana Bread

Apple Crisp

Vanilla Cream Oatmeal

Chocolate Cookie Oatmeal

Protein Granola Yogurt

Blueberry Coconut Omelet

Banana Split Protein Oats

French Toast

Sausage and Egg Bell Pepper Breakfast

Stuffed Baked Breakfast Apple

Tomato Basil Omelet

Spicy Scrambled Eggs

Protein Pancakes

Serves: 6
Preparation time: 20 minutes
Cooking time: 15 minutes

Ingredients:

½ Banana mashed
½ cup (125ml) liquid Egg Whites
1 Tbsp. (15ml) Chia seeds
1 cup (250ml) organic quick Oats
1 scoop Peanut Butter flavored Whey Protein
½ cup (125ml) Almond Milk
½ cup (125ml) Water
Pinch of salt

Method:

Mix all the ingredients together in a large bowl, until well blended – you can use a hand mixer or blender for this as well.

Let the mixture sit for 10-15 minutes, allowing for the gluten to develop and the Chia seeds to expand, which will make your pancakes come out fluffier.

Heat a medium sized pan and coat with non-stick cooking spray.
Keep the heat on medium to thoroughly cook pancakes.
Use 1/3 cup (85ml) measuring cup and pour the mixture into the pan.

These pancakes take about 1½– 2 minutes on each side to cook.

Recommended Toppings:

Vanilla Greek Yogurt
Blueberries

Macronutrients: (per pancake)

Protein: 10g
Carbs: 12g
Fat: 2g

Calories: 66

Oatmeal & Egg Whites

Serves: 1
Preparation time: 5 minutes
Cooking time:5 minutes

Ingredients:

1½ oz (40g) Oatmeal
½ cup (125ml) Non-Fat Milk
1 tsp (5ml) Peanut Butter
1 tsp (5ml) 85% Dark Chocolate, chopped or grated
Pinch of Salt

On the side:
3 Egg Whites
½ slice of Non-Fat Cheese

Method:

Place the oats in a medium sized bowl, add the milk and cook it in the microwave on high for about 1½ minutes. Add the peanut butter and chocolate, stir well.

Heat a frying pan over a medium heat and coat with a non-stick spray, add eggs and cook.
Place on a plate, add the cheese and mix for flavor

Macronutrients:

Protein: 25g
Carbs: 37g
Fat: 8g

Calories: 316

Light Breakfast

Serves: 1
Preparation time: 5 Minutes
Cooking time: none

Ingredients:

170g Chobani Greek Yogurt
2 heaped Tbsp (40ml) Jordan's Super Berry Granola
1 Banana chopped or mashed / alternatively ¼ cup (65ml) Blueberries
1 scoop Vanilla Whey Protein

Method:

Mix the whey powder and yogurt first, add the granola and banana and mix well.

Macronutrients:

Protein: 47g
Carbs: 10g
Fat: 2g

Calories 246

Serves: 1
Preparation time: 5 Minutes
Cooking time: 5 Minutes

Ingredients:

2 whole Eggs
2 Egg Whites
20g Spelt Flakes
Chives, chopped
Pinch of Salt
Pepper to taste

Method:

Mix whole eggs and egg whites in a cup and flavor with salt and pepper to taste.
Heat a medium size frying pan and coat with nonstick spray.
Cook the eggs, and add the spelt flakes.
Garnish with chives and serve.

Macronutrients:

Protein: 34g
Carbs: 14g
Fats: 13g

Calories: 310

Serves: 1
Preparation time: 5 minutes
Cooking time: 15 minutes

Ingredients:

6 Egg Whites
1 Egg Yolk
30g Fat-Free Cheddar Cheese, shredded
2 Fat-Free flour Tortillas
Salt to taste

Method:

Place the tortillas on a baking tray or plate.
Place eggs and yolk in a mixing bowl and beat well.
Heat the tortillas in either the microwave or oven.
Heat a skillet and coat with nonstick cooking spray. Cook
the eggs over a medium flame, turn over and add the
cheese.
Place eggs in tortillas and serve.

Additions:

Salsa
Parsley or chopped spring onion

Macronutrients:

Protein: 15g
Carbs: 16g
Fat: 0.5g

Calories:131

Big Breakfast Pizza
Servings: 1
Preparation time: 10 minutes
Cooking time: 10 minutes

Ingredients:

2 slices Jennie-O extra-lean Turkey Bacon. Alternatively, 1
turkey sausage patty
3 whole Eggs
¼ Boboli 12" thin Pizza Crust
½ cup (62ml) Fat-Free Mozzarella or Cheddar cheese
¼ small Onion, diced
½ Tomato, diced
Hot sauce (optional)
Salt and pepper to taste

Method:

If you are using turkey bacon, place bacon on a plate
between two paper towels and microwave for one
minute.
Flip bacon over, keeping it in the paper towels and
remove the top paper towel. Place a new paper towel on

top, and microwave for another minute.

Remove from microwave and cut into 1 inch pieces.

If making with turkey sausage, cook according to package instructions then cut into small pieces.

Place the pizza crust on a baking sheet and heat in a toaster oven.

Place the eggs in a mixing bowl, season with salt and pepper to taste, and beat well.

Heat a skillet and coat with a nonstick cooking spray.

Sauté the onions and add the tomatoes. Add your choice of meat to the pan, and allow to simmer for a few minutes.

Add the beaten eggs and mix well. Add the hot sauce and remove from the heat.

Place the mixture on the heated pizza base and serve.

Tasty Additions:

Chopped spring onion

Chopped garlic

2 Chopped or sliced Mushrooms

Macronutrients:

Protein: 40g

Carbs: 49g

Fat: 22g

Calories: 575

Vanilla Protein Porridge

Servings: 1
Preparation time: 5 minutes
Cooking time: 2 minutes

Ingredients:

1 cup (250 ml) Oats
½ cup (125ml) Skim Milk
1 scoop Vanilla Protein whey (for variation, try other flavors)
½ tsp (2,5ml) Stevia or 1 Tbsp (15ml) Honey
Salt and Cinnamon to taste

Tasty Additions:

Mixed Berries or Blueberries

Method:

Place the oats, skim milk, stevia, salt, cinnamon and fruit in a microwave safe mixing bowl. Mix well and place in the microwave for 1 minute on high remove, stir and repeat. Remove and stir in the protein whey. Serve hot.

Macronutrients:

Protein: 45g
Carbs: 45g
Fat: 5g

Calories: 404

Chocolate Peanut Butter & Banana Oatmeal

Serves: 1
Preparation time: 5 Minutes
Cooking time: 2 Minutes

Ingredients:

1/2 cup (125ml) Oats
1/2 cup (125ml) Almond Milk
1 Banana, mashed
1 scoop Chocolate Peanut Butter Protein Powder
Pinch of Salt

Method:

Place the banana and milk in a mixing bowl and mix well.
Add the oats and mix.
Add ½ cup water, and mix.
Microwave for 2 minutes on high heat.
Remove and stir in the protein powder
Microwave for 1 more minute or longer for the
consistency you like.

Macronutrients:

Protein: 33g
Carbs: 68g
Fat: 6g

Calories: 416

Apple Cinnamon Oatmeal

Serves: 1
Preparation time: 3 minutes
Cooking time: 3 minutes

Ingredients:

1 cup (250ml) rolled or steel cut Oats
½ cup (125ml) Water
½ an Apple, cut into small pieces
½ tsp (2,5ml) Cinnamon
1 scoop Vanilla Whey Protein
Pinch of Salt

Method:

Place the oats, apple, cinnamon, salt and water in a microwave safe mixing bowl, and mix well.
Microwave for 1 minutes on high heat, remove and stir then microwave for 1 more minute
Remove.
Mix in 1 scoop of vanilla whey protein.
Serve hot.

Macronutrients:

Protein: 30g
Carbs: 45g
Fat; 6g

Calories: 354

Peanut Butter, Banana Oat Breakfast Cookies

Servings: 16
Preparation time: 20 minutes
Cooking time: 30 minutes

Ingredients:

2 ripe Bananas, mashed until smooth & creamy
⅓ cup (85ml) Peanut Butter ~ creamy or chunky
⅔ cup (200ml) unsweetened Applesauce
1 scoop Vanilla Protein Powder
1 tsp (5ml) Vanilla Extract
1½ cups (375ml) Quick Cooking Oatmeal
¼ cup (63ml) chopped Nuts

Method:

Preheat heat oven to 350 F (180 C)
In a large bowl, mix mashed banana & peanut butter until completely combined then add in the applesauce, vanilla protein powder & the extract ~ mix again until all are completely combined.
Add in the oatmeal & nuts to the banana mixture & combine.
Let dough rest for 10 minutes.
Drop cookie dough, by spoonfuls, onto a parchment paper lined cookie sheet & flatten cookies into circles.
Bake cookies for 20-30 minutes, or until golden brown & done.

Macronutrients:

Protein: 4.5g
Carbs: 11.5g
Fat: 4.5g

Calories: 99

2 Minute Pancakes

Serves: 1
Preparation time: 5 minutes
Cooking time: 2 minutes

Ingredients:

4 Egg Whites.
1 scoop Chocolate Flavored Whey
45g Oats.

Method:

Mix in a bowl until you have a thick slurpy liquid.
Heat a skillet over a medium flame and Spray with a
nonstick spray. Pour the mixture into the pan

Toppings

Yogurt
Fresh cut Fruit
Peanut Butter

Macronutrients:

Protein: 39g
Carbs: 35g
Fat: 3g

Calories: 323

French Toast Cups
Servings: 1
Preparation time: 5 minutes
Cooking time: 15 minutes

Ingredients:

2 eggs, or ½ cup (125ml) Egg Whites
1-2 tsp (10ml) Stevia
½ tsp (2,5ml) Vanilla Extract
¼ tsp (2ml) Cinnamon
Sea salt to taste
2 slices Wholegrain Bread
½ cup (125ml) Low-Fat Cottage Cheese

Method:

Preheat oven to 350 F (180 C).
In a shallow bowl, combine eggs, I tsp (5ml) Stevie, vanilla
extract, a dash of cinnamon and salt, as desired. Dip
bread slices into egg mixture, soaking thoroughly.

Spray 2 cups in a muffin tin with nonstick spray. Gently press one piece of bread into each cup. Press down to make sure they nearly touch the bottom of the pan. Place muffin tin in oven and bake for 15 minutes.

In a separate bowl, mix the cottage cheese with remaining Stevia and cinnamon. Top each French toast cup with half of the mixture and serve hot.

Macronutrients:

Protein: 34g
Carbs: 28g
Fat:16g

Calories: 390

Mocha Oatmeal

Servings: 1
Preparation time: 5 minutes
Cooking time: 20 minutes

Ingredients:

1 cup (250ml) premade Instant Coffee
½ cup (125ml) Oatmeal
½ cup (125ml) Cottage Cheese
1 Tbsp. (15ml) unsweetened Cacao
½ cup (125ml) 1% Chocolate Milk

Method:

Cook oatmeal in the coffee for 15 minutes on the stovetop.
Add in the cottage cheese and the cacao and cook for another 5 minutes.
During the very last 2 minutes pour in the chocolate milk.
Add splenda or other sweetener if needed.

Macronutrients:

Protein: 27g
Carbs: 56g
Fat: 7g

Calories: 395

Banana Bread

Servings: 5
Preparation time: 10 minutes
Cooking time: 35 minutes

Ingredients:

1 cup (250ml) Oatmeal
2 small Bananas, mashed
1 Egg
½ cup (125 ml) Skim Milk
2 tsp (10ml) Cinnamon
100g Low Fat Cottage Cheese
1 heaped scoop of Banana or Vanilla Flavored Whey
Protein (about 40 grams)
1 tsp (5ml) Baking Powder

Method:

Preheat the oven to 350 F (180 C).
Spray a small bread-loaf tin with a nonstick spray.
Mix all the ingredients together, and pour into a baking
tin.
Bake for 35 minutes until golden brown.
Serve cooled.

Macronutrients (per serving):

Protein: 13g
Carbs: 23g
Fat: 4g

Calories: 191

Apple Crisp

Servings: 1
Preparation time: 10 minutes
Cooking time: None

Ingredients:

½ cup (125ml) rolled Oats
1 cup (250ml) Kashi GoLean cereal
10-15 Raisins
1 Tbsp (15ml) Honey
½ Tbsp (7,5ml) Cinnamon or to taste
1 small Granny Smith or Golden Delicious Apple, diced finely
150ml Water

Method:

Place everything in a mixing bowl and mix before adding the water (a little more if you want) Mix well and consume immediately.

Macronutrients:

Protein: 19g
Carbs: 92g
Fat: 4g

Calories: 420

Vanilla Cream Oatmeal

Servings: 1
Preparation time: 7 minutes
Cooking time: 2 minutes

Ingredients:

1 cup (250ml) Oatmeal
1cup (250ml) Skim Milk
1 scoop (30g) Vanilla Protein Powder
½ tsp (2,5ml) of Stevia
Pinch of Cinnamon
Pinch of Salt

Method:

In a microwave proof mixing bowl, add the salt, oatmeal
skim milk and cinnamon, mix well. Place in the microwave
and cook at full power for about 1 minute - stir the mix ,
then microwave for another 1 minute period.
Let the oatmeal cool for about 3 minutes add the Stevia
and protein powder.

Consume immediately.

Macronutrients:

Protein: 45g
Carbs: 73g
Fat: 6g

Calories: 531

Chocolate Cookie Oatmeal

Servings: 1
Preparation time: 5 minutes
Cooking time: None

Ingredients:

½ cup (125ml) uncooked Oats
1 Tbsp (15ml) natural Peanut Butter
1 scoop (40g) Chocolate Whey Powder
4 Tbsp (60ml) boiling Water
2 packets Splenda

Method:

Add water to oats, and let it stand for 30 seconds.
Add whey, splenda and peanut butter, and mix well.
Consume immediately.

Macronutrients:

Protein: 31g
Carbs: 32g
Fat: 12g

Calories: 370

Protein Granola Yogurt

Servings: 1

Preparation time: 20 minutes

Cooking time: None

Ingredients:

¾ cup (180ml) Fat Free Greek Yogurt

1 Scoop (30g) Vanilla Protein Powder

1 Tbsp (15ml) Chia Seeds

2 Tbsp (30ml) Granola/Granola Type Cereal

⅔ cup (100g) chopped Strawberries

Alternative fruits:

Blueberries

Cranberries

Apple

Method:

Place all the ingredients except the fruit in a small mixing or serving bowl and mix well. Allow to stand for 15-20 minutes, to allow the chia seeds to swell and the granola to soften.

Add the fruit, mix and enjoy.

Tips:

This yogurt can be frozen, and consumed as a filling treat on a warm day.

Macronutrients:

Protein: 46g
Carbs: 52g
Fat: 5g

Calories: 437

Blueberry Coconut Omelet
Serves: 1
Preparation time: 10 minutes
Cooking time: 5 minutes

Ingredients:

1 tsp (5ml) Coconut Oil
½ cup (125ml) liquid Egg Whites
¼ tsp (2ml) Vanilla Extract
Pinch of Salt
½ tsp (2,5ml) Sweetener or Stevia
⅓ cup (85ml) thawed or fresh Blueberries
1 Tbsp (15ml) desiccated or shredded Coconut
½ Tbsp (7,5ml) White Chocolate Peanut Butter

Method:

Combine the egg whites, salt, vanilla &
sweetener/cinnamon in a small mixing bowl and mix.
Well
Heat a small frying pan over medium heat and add the
coconut oil.

Once the pan is hot, pour in the mixture. As the mixture starts to set add your blueberries & coconut to one half, and cook for another minute or so, before flipping.
Cook for another minute, flip the omelet one last time onto its other side, and cook until golden brown and add the peanut butter to the top of the omelet.

Fold the omelet and serve immediately.

Nutrition Facts:

Protein: 15g
Carbs: 13g
Fat: 11g

Calories: 208

Banana Split Protein Oats

Serves: 1
Preparation time: Overnight
Cooking time: None

Ingredients:

1 cup (250ml) Blue Diamond Almond Breeze
Unsweetened Vanilla Milk
1 scoop (30g) BSN Syntha-6 Peanut Butter Protein
Powder
1 small Banana
½ cup (125ml) dry Quaker Old Fashioned Oats
¼ cup Almond Milk
4 tsp (20ml) Walden Farms Sugar Free Calorie Free
Chocolate Syrup
2 packets Stevia Sweetener
Chopped Nuts, (optional)

Method:

In a small mixing bowl combine the oats, Sythna, peanut
butter cookie protein powder, stevia, and almond milk,
and allow to swell overnight

The following morning, cut the banana in half lengthwise,
and place in a dish.
Put the oat mix in between the banana halves
Top with Walden Farms Chocolate Syrup, and chopped
nuts.

Macronutrients:

Protein: 30g
Carbs: 64g
Fat: 12g

Calories: 470

French Toast
Serves: 3
Preparation time: 5 minutes
Cooking time: 5 minutes

Ingredients:

6 slices Sara lee Delightful Whole Wheat and Honey 45
calorie bread
250g Egg Whites
½ cup (125ml) unsweetened Almond Milk
2 packets sweetener or Stevia
½ tsp (2ml) Baking Powder/Baking Soda

Method:

Preheat a pancake griddle at a medium heat
Combine the egg whites, almond milk, baking powder,
and sweetener in a shallow dish
Using two forks, place each slice of bread in the egg
mixture, turning over to saturate both sides.
Place each slice on the griddle and cook until a golden
color is achieved, turn and repeat.

Top with your favorite syrup or jam, but remember to adjust the macros!

Tips:

Use a medium high heat if you desire a more moist toast, as the outside will be done prior to drying out the inside.

Also for a more moist toast, decrease the amount of egg whites and/or increase the amount of almond milk. Vice versa for a crispier toast. The amount of necessary egg whites may vary by the bread you use. The Sara Lee bread absorbs liquid like a sponge!

Macronutrients (per serving):

Protein: 46g
Carbs: 43
Fat: 4g

Calories: 423

Sausage and Egg Bell Pepper Breakfast

Serves: 1

Preparation time: 15 minutes

Cooking time: 10 minutes

Ingredients:

1 medium Publix Red Bell Pepper

2 large Egg Whites

½ cup (125ml) cooked Turkey Breakfast Sausage

2 Tbsp (10g) Cheddar or American Cheese (Reduced Fat, Pasteurized)

⅔ tsp (4ml) Parsley

Method:

Preheat the oven to 400 F (220 C)

Prepare 90% lean turkey breakfast sausage in advance.

Cut the top off a bell pepper and place into an oven (directly on the rack) at for 10 minutes.

Scramble 2 egg whites in a pan. Combine with your prepared turkey sausage. Mix in the shredded reduced fat cheddar cheese. Stuff into finished bell pepper and top with parsley or green onions.

Macronutrients:

Protein: 27g

Carbs: 9g

Fat: 7g

Calories: 212

Stuffed Baked Breakfast Apple

Serves: 3
Preparation time: 10 minutes
Cooking time: 10 minutes

Ingredients:

3 Granny Smith of Golden Delicious Apples, cored and pitted
1½ cups (375ml) Non-fat Greek Yogurt
1 scoop (30g) Vanilla Protein Powder
½ cup (125ml) rolled Oats
3 Tbsp (45ml) chopped Walnuts
1 tsp (5ml) Cinnamon
2 Tbsp (30ml) Splenda Brown Sugar Blend

Method:

Combine the cinnamon and brown sugar.
Place the cored apple in the mixture. Coat the apple, inside and out, and place on the grill.
Cook for 3-4 minutes or until tender.
Mix the Greek yogurt, protein powder, rolled oats, and walnuts until well mixed.
Fill the baked apple with the mixture.

Cover and cook for 1-2 minutes or until yogurt is heated.

Macronutrients:

Protein:25 g
Carbs: 50g
Fat: 11g

Calories: 393

Tomato Basil Omelet
Serves: 1
Preparation time: 5 minutes
Cooking time: 5 minutes

Ingredients:

3 free range Eggs
10 Cherry Tomatoes
Fresh Basil
Sea Salt
Black Pepper
Kelp
1 Tbsp (15ml) Palm Oil, for cooking

Method:

In a mixing bowl, whisk 3 whole eggs with salt, pepper, basil, and kelp.
Slice 10 cherry tomatoes.
Coat skillet with palm oil.
Pour everything into the skillet and cook over medium heat.

If you add sausage, brown it in a separate pan before adding it to the omelet.

Flip once. When done fold and serve immediately.

Macronutrients:

Protein: 10g
Carbs: 12g
Fat: 11g

Calories: 186

Spicy Scrambled Eggs

Serves: 1
Preparation time: 5 minutes
Cooking time: 5 minutes

Ingredients:

2 large Whole Eggs
4 Eggs Whites
¼ of an Onion, finely chopped
1 whole red Chili (or chili to taste), finely chopped
1 clove Garlic, finely chopped
50g Cottage Cheese
Pinch of Mixed Herbs
2 slices of whole Brown Bread

Method:

In a small mixing bowl combine the whole eggs and egg whites. Whisk until the egg yolks and whites mix.

To this, add the chopped onion, garlic and chili, mix well. Finally, add the cottage cheese and a pinch of mixed herbs, Whisk.

Heat a small non-stick frying pan over a medium flame, coat with a non-stick spray.

Empty the contents of the mixing bowl into the frying pan.

Put your toast in the toaster. Gently stir the contents to scramble the eggs

Once eggs are scrambled, add them to toast on a large plate.

Macronutrients:

Protein: 50g
Carbs: 34g
Fat: 19g

Calories: 507

Main Meals

Thai Spiced Chicken Beef and Basil

High Protein BBQ Chicken Pizza

Turkey Chili Frito Pie

Flavorsome Chicken Stir fry

Egg 'n Tuna

Tortilla Pizza

High Protein Sandwiches

Asian Wok

No-nonsense Chicken Noodles

Chicken Pad Thai

Steamed Hamburgers with Sweet Potato Fries

Spicy Pasta

Butternut Lasagne

Chilli Con Turkey

Turkey Burgers

Chicken Cordon Bleu

Lean Turkey Meatloaf

Salsa Chicken Tortilla

Bistro-Style White Bean Burger with Fried Egg and Avocado

Couscous Salad with Tuna and Avocado

Herb Garden Beef Burger

Beef and Rice Mash

Avocado Lime Chicken

Marinated Chicken Enchiladas

Spanish Rice

Asian Flank Steak and Stir-Fry

Protein Pumpkin Pie

Baked Chicken

Turkey Power Balls

Honey Nut Barbeque Chicken Fingers

Chicken Egg White Pizza

Curry Rice

Salmon Balls

Peanut Butter Chicken

Baked Pineapple Chicken

Slow Cooked Chicken Stew

Italian Slow Cooked Chicken

Sloppy Joes

Creamy Artichoke Chicken

Spicy Coconut Chicken Tenders

Peanut Butter Chicken

Chicken Avocado Burger Patties

Tuna Melt

Chicken Pot Pie

Spicy Chicken Lentils

Spicy Turkey Chili

Rotisserie Chicken Noodle Pasta Bake

Teriyaki Salmon

Field of Greens

Lobster Boat

Spicy Turkey Meatballs

Chicken Cheese Meatballs

Chicken Caesar Meatballs

Fish in Foil

Chicken Cucumber Salad

Sweet Potato Omelet

Thai Spicy Beef Salad

Malaysian Curry Prawns

Chicken Curry

Beef Chop Suey

Salsa Quinoa Chicken

Grilled Tuna Burgers

Tuna Cheese Melt

Beef and Basil

Serves: 1
Preparation time: 5 minutes
Cooking time: 5 minutes

Ingredients:

Spinach
Corn
Baby Tomatoes
Mushrooms
Minced Fresh Basil
Eggs
Lean Sirloin Steak (150g - 200g)

Method:

Begin by boiling 1 egg.
Warm a pan with some olive oil. Thrown in handful of corn and halved baby tomatoes.
Stir fry for a little, and add some minced basil.
Add your sliced mushrooms.
Prep your salad bowl with spinach as the base.
Once the corn, tomato and mushroom mixture is basiled up
Heat a little oil in a pan and place the sirloin steak in. A little of salt and pepper on the uncooked side is enough for seasoning.
After a couple of minutes, flip the meat.
Place the meat on a plate and rest for a further 3-5minutes to ensure the juices redistribute throughout the meat. Peel the egg and mash up in a small bowl.

Place a mound of the spinach, corn,tomato and mushroom salad on a plate.
Place thin slices of the sirloin on top
Grab the egg mixture and place a thin strip of it on top of the steak.

Macronutrients: (per serve)

Protein: 57 Grams
Carbs: 23 Grams
Fat: 15 Grams

Calories: 463

Serves: 8
Preparation time: 10 minutes
Cooking time: 20 minutes

Ingredients:

1 Whole Boboli Whole Wheat Thin Pizza Crust
3 servings (90g) 2% Mozzarella shredded cheese
13oz (850g) boneless Chicken Breast
½ Tbsp (7,5ml) Olive Oil
2.5oz (74ml) chopped Onions
2 servings (60ml) BBQ Sauce

Method:

Preheat a skillet on a medium-high flame, and your oven
to 450 F (220 C)
Chop chicken and onions
Pour olive oil in preheated skillet
Place chicken and onions in skillet, stir so olive oil coats
the chicken/onions. Season and cook thoroughly
Open Boboli pizza crust and baste with BBQ sauce
Place the cooked chicken on pizza crust and cover with
cheese
Cook in oven for 12 minutes

Macronutrients: (per serve)

Protein: 20g
Carbs: 20g
Fat: 5g

Calories: 210

Turkey Chili Frito Pie

Serves: 1
Preparation time: 5 minutes
Cooking time: 5 minutes

Ingredients:

1 can Wolf Brand Turkey Chili.
60g 2% Milk Shredded Cheese
30g of plain Fritos

Method:

Empty the contents of the tin into a microwave proof bowl.
Place in microwave and cook at full power for a minute and a half.
Remove the bowl and stir well.
Sprinkle the cheese on top and return to the microwave for a minute,
Add 1 serving of plain Fritos and stir.

Serve immediately.

Macronutrients:

Protein: 71g
Carbs: 47.5g
Fats 33g

Calories: 771

Flavorsome Chicken Stir fry

Serves: 1
Preparation time: 5 minutes
Cooking time: 35 minutes

Ingredients:

150g Chicken, cut in strips
100g Broccoli broken up
2 slices of Pineapple cut into chunks
1 tsp (5ml) Soy Sauce
1 tsp (5ml) Olive Oil
100g uncooked Brown rice

Method:

Boil the brown rice.
Heat a wok and add a small amount of water with the olive oil.
Place the broccoli in the middle and cook for 5 minutes.
Move the broccoli to the outsides and add the chicken, and fry for 2 minutes.

Mix the broccoli and chicken then add the pineapple and soy sauce, and cook for 2 minutes.
Add the cooked rice to the wok and mix.
Add seasoning (hot sauce), if desired

Macronutrients:

Protein: 47g
Carbs: 70g
Fats: 14g

Calories: 585

Egg 'n Tuna

Serves: 1
Preparation time: 5 minutes
Cooking time: 5 minutes

Ingredients:

135g (1 can) Tuna,
2 Whole Eggs
100g of Cottage Cheese
20g of Cheese

Method:

Heat a small frying pan, and coat it with a nonstick spray.
Open and drain the tuna, and add to the pan, cook for
two minutes.
Add the cottage cheese, and mix well.
Add salt and pepper to taste.
Shell the two eggs and beat lightly, then add to the
mixture.
Cook until eggs are done.
Add the cheese and cheese, and serve immediately.

Macronutrients:

Protein: 66g
Carbs: 2g
Fats: 19g

Calories: 443

Tortilla Pizza

Serves: 1
Preparation time: 5 minutes
Cooking time: 10 minutes

Ingredients:

1 Plain tortilla
40g Low-Fat Mozzarella
⅓ jar Napolina Pizza Sauce
200g Chicken Breast, cut in strips or cubes

Method:

Heat a small skillet and spray with nonstick spray,
Cook the chicken, add seasoning if desired.

Lay tortilla flat and spread the pizza sauce over it, and
sprinkle with the cheese.
Add the chicken and place under the grill until the cheese
has melted.

Serve immediately

Macronutrients:

Protein: 62g
Carbs: 40g
Fats: 12g

Calories: 516

Serves: 1
Preparation time: 5 minutes
Cooking time: 5 minutes

Ingredients:

5 large Egg Whites
2 Bread
1 Tbsp (15ml) Olive oil
4 Tbsp 60ml Cheddar cheese
Salt and Pepper to taste

Method:

Heat a medium sized skillet over a low-medium flame and add the olive oil.
Add the egg whites into the pan and cook for two minutes or until whites have set.
Sprinkle the cheddar cheese onto egg, and allow to melt.
Season with salt and pepper.
Fold the egg first in half then in quarters and place in a slice of bread
Season with sauce if so desired
Cover with another slice and serve immediately.

Macronutrients:

Protein: 30g
Carbs: 31g
Fats: 7g

Calories: 307

Asian Wok

Serves: 1
Preparation time: 10 minutes
Cooking time: 30 minutes

Ingredients:

150g Chicken cut into strips
100g Basmati rice
50g Zucchini grated
½ tsp (2.5ml) Paprika
2 tsp (10ml) Wok sauce
Curry Powder

Method:

Boil the rice according to cooking directions.
Heat a wok and add a small amount of water with the olive oil.
Place the Zucchini in the middle and cook for 2 minutes.
Move the Zucchini to the outsides and add the chicken, and fry for 5 minutes.
Mix the Zucchini and chicken then add the paprika, curry powder and wok sauce, and cook for 2 minutes.
Add the cooked rice to the wok and mix.
Add seasoning (hot sauce), if desired.

Macronutrients:

Protein: 43g
Carbs: 84g
Fats: 4g

Calories: 528

No-nonsense Chicken Noodles
Serves: 1
Preparation time: 5 minutes
Cooking time: 5 minutes

Ingredients:

100g egg noodles
250g chicken breast cut in strips
Chili sauce to taste
Worcester sauce to taste
Tikka powder to taste

Method:

Boil 100g egg noodles,
Heat a medium sized frying pan once a medium high
flame and coat with nonstick spray.
Add chicken and cook,
When chicken is almost cooked, add chili sauce,
Worcester sauce and tikka powder, lower the heat and
allow to simmer.
Brain the noodles and place in a bowl, season with
Worcester sauce if desired.
Place chicken on noodles.

Serve immediately

Macronutrients:

Protein: 80g
Carbs: 60g
Fats: 10g

Calories: 540

Chicken Pad Thai
Serves: 1
Preparation time: 5 minutes
Cooking time: 10 minutes

Ingredients:

2 cups (500ml) cooked Whole Wheat Angel Hair Pasta
3.3oz. (95g) Chicken Breasts, cut into bite sized pieces
1 cup (250ml) sliced Mushrooms
½ cup (125l) sliced Yellow Pepper
1 Tbsp (15ml) Fish Sauce
¼ cup (63ml)chopped cilantro
1 tsp (5ml) olive oil
1 Tbsp (15ml)natural peanut butter
1 Tbsp. (15ml) Splenda (3packets)
1 Tbsp. red Chili Flakes

Method:

Prepare the pasta according to package directions.
Heat the oil in a skillet over medium heat, and add the
chicken, cook for 2-3 minutes.

Add the peppers and mushrooms and cook for another 3-5 minutes or until chicken is fully cooked.

Mix the fish sauce, peanut butter, Splenda, and chili flakes and pour over the chicken.

Cover, and simmer for 3-4 minutes.

Top with cilantro before serving.

Macronutrients:

Protein: 56g
Carbs: 39g
Fat: 14g

Calories: 458

Steamed Hamburgers with Sweet Potato Fries

Serves: 1
Preparation time: 10 minutes
Cooking time: 25 minutes

Ingredients:

1 Chicken Filet (about 150-200 grams)
2 Whole Wheat Hamburger Buns
Lettuce, Cucumber, Tomato, Onion as garnish
2 Sweet Potatoes
1 tsp (5ml) Olive Oil
Salt, Pepper, Basil
1 big Tomato

Method:

Preheat the oven to 450 F (230 C).
Put the chicken fillet through the meat grinder and season it.
Cut French fries of your sweet potatoes, add one teaspoon of olive oil and season it with a pinch of salt, pepper and garlic.
Divide the chicken and place the meat in empty tuna cans and place in a steamer. Set a timer for about 15-20 minutes.
Insert potatoes in the oven. After 10-15 minutes, turn the fries so they can become crispy on both sides.
Garnish the hamburger buns with some lettuce, tomato, cucumber, onion.
Finish it off with the hamburgers and some dressing of your choice.

Macronutrients:

Proteins: 56g
Carbs: 152g
Fats: 5g

Calories: 806

Spicy Pasta
Serves: 1
Preparation time: 5 minutes
Cooking time: 15 minutes

Ingredients:

2 Trader Joe's Spicy Italian Chicken Sausages
4 oz (120g) Ground Beef
4oz (120g) boneless, skinless Chicken Breast
1 cup (250ml) Whole Wheat Penne
Fresh Basil
Garlic, chopped or crushed
2 Tbsp (15ml) EVOO
2 Tomatoes, chopped

Method:

Cook paste as per package instructions.

Heat a medium sized frying pan and add the beef chicken tomatoes and cook them together. Add the sausages, and allow to simmer over a low hat for 5-10 minutes.

Add some freshly chopped garlic and basil, and cook until basil has wilted.

Drain pasta and place on plate, spoon the meat over and garnish with EVVO.

Serve immediately.

acronutrients:

Protein: 103g
Carbs: 126g
Fat: 59g

Calories: 1,430

Butternut Lasagna

Serves: 4

Preparation time: 20 minutes

Cooking time: 95 minutes

Ingredients:

1½ lbs (620g) Butternut Squash, cut and deseeded

3.5 oz (100g) Lasagna Noodles (sheets)

500g Cottage or Ricotta Cheese

5 cups (1.25ℓ) Spinach, chopped

50g shredded Cheese

Sauce:

2 cups (500ml) Milk

3 Tbsp (45ml) Flour

Method:

Cook the butternut squash:

Preheat oven to 450 F (230 C).

Split butternut in half. Place in baking dish and fill about 1inch (2,5cm) of water. Place in oven and bake for 40 minutes, until tender. Scoop out flesh and discard skin, mash the flesh.

Adjust oven to 350 F (180 C)

Filling: Wilt spinach in a pan, then cool and add 500g cottage cheese and stir.

Sauce: Heat up milk in small saucepan on low heat. Whisk in small amounts of flour; roughly ½ teaspoon at a time. Once all flour has been mixed in, bring up to a boil, whisking continuously. Once the sauce thickens, turn heat off (use immediately).

Once the squash, filling, and sauce are finished, you are ready to start building your dish.

Use cooking spray or a light swipe of cooking oil to cover a 9 x 13 cooking dish. Use 1 cup of the sauce to cover the entire bottom of the dish. Place a layer of (cooked or uncooked) noodles side by side to make the next layer of the lasagna, use half of the ricotta/cottage cheese and spinach mixture to cover the noodles.
Next, layer all of the roasted butternut squash, followed by the last half of the ricotta/cottage cheese spinach filling. Top with another layer of lasagna noodles, then cover those with the remaining sauce and the grated cheese.

Cover the Butternut Squash Lasagna with tin foil and bake at for 40 minutes. Uncover and cook for another 15 minutes. Let it cool for 5 minutes before serving.

Macronutrients (per serve):
Protein: 101g
Carb: 201g
Fat: 30g
Calories: 1,470

Chili Con Turkey

Serves: 4
Preparation time: 5 minutes
Cooking time: 5 minutes

Ingredients:

450g ground Turkey
1 can Mexican style diced Tomatoes
1 can Black Beans, rinsed and drained
1 can whole-kernel Sweet Corn, drained
1 package dried Chili mix
1 Tbsp (15ml) Ground Flaxseed
1/4 cup (63ml) Water
1 cup (250ml) cooked Rice

Method:

Brown the turkey in a skillet over medium high heat
Add everything else but the rice and cook over low heat
for 10 minutes.
Serve over rice

Macronutrients (per serve):

Protein: 30g
Carbs: 52g
Fats: 11g

Calories: 407

Turkey Burgers

Serves: 1
Preparation time: 10 minutes
Cooking time: 30 minutes

Ingredients:

125g of Turkey Breast mince
¼ cup (63ml) of finely diced Onion
¼ cup (63ml) of finely diced Red Pepper
1 Garlic clove, peeled and minced
¼ tsp (1ml) ground Black Pepper
2 tsp (10ml) of Olive Oil

Method:

Preheat your oven to 350 F (180 C)
Add the diced red pepper, diced onion, minced garlic, turkey breast mince to a mixing bowl. Add the olive oil and the ground black pepper. Mix well and add any spices if you would like to enhance the flavor.
Form two patties and place on the grill.
Cook the patties in the oven for13 minutes. Then turn over and cook for another 13 minutes.
Serve with whole-meal teacakes, lettuce, tomato and onion.

Macronutrients:

Protein: 39.5 g
Carbs: 13.3 g
Fats: 2.6 g

Calories: 175.8

Chicken Cordon Bleu

Serves: 2
Preparation time: 10 minutes
Cooking time: 30 minutes

Ingredients:

4oz (120g) boneless skinless Chicken Breasts
8 Kirkland Honey Smoked Ham slices
½ cup (125ml) Reduced-Fat shredded Mozzarella
Salt, Pepper and Garlic seasoning to taste
1 cup (250ml)-mashed Sweet Potato
6 oz (170g) Kirkland stir-fry frozen vegetables
4 Ritz Crackers, crushed.

Method:

Pre-heat oven to 375 F (200 C)
Pound the chicken breast to ¼ inch (6mm) thickness.
Season both sides with salt, pepper, garlic powder, place
2 slices of ham on top of breasts, Sprinkle with shredded
mozzarella and roll up,
Sprinkle the top of the rolls with crushed ritz crackers.

Bake in oven for 25-30 minutes at 375.

Wash and peel sweet potatoes. Cube the potatoes and
steam boil potatoes for about 25 minutes.

Place 6 oz of frozen veggies in small saucepan, boil with ¼
cup water and season to taste.

Macronutrients (per serve):

Protein: 38g
Carbs: 60g
Fats: 12g

Calories: 443

Lean Turkey Meatloaf
Serves: 2
Preparation time: 10 minutes
Cooking time: 50 minutes

Ingredients:

1lb (450g) of Ground Turkey
½ can of Tomato Sauce
2 whole Eggs
1 cup (250ml) of Whole-Wheat Breadcrumbs
½ Onion, diced.
Seasoning and Salt to your taste.

Method:

Preheat oven to 375 F (180 C)

Mix all ingredients together in a bowl, place the mixture
in a baking tray lined with foil, shape into a loaf, bake for
45 minutes.

Top with shrircha hot sauce and a little BBQ sauce, then place in oven for another 15 minutes

Macronutrients:

Protein: 28g
Carbs: 18g
Fats: 4g

Calories: 220

Salsa Chicken Tortilla
Serves: 1
Preparation time: 5 minutes
Cooking time: 10 minutes

Ingredients:

¾ cup (190 ml) diced precooked Chicken
2 Tbsp (30ml) diced Onion
2 Tbsp (30ml) Feta-Cheese crumbles
1 handful romaine lettuce, chopped
1 large whole-wheat tortilla
Salsa for dipping

Method:

Arrange the chicken, onion, cheese, and lettuce down the center of the tortilla.
Roll it tightly and cut it in half.
Grill the rolls seam-side down for 2 to 3 minutes per side, on a nonstick skillet heated to medium.

Serve with salsa. Makes 1 serving

Macronutrients:

Protein: 56g
Carbs: 10g
Fats: 10g

Calories: 397

Bistro-Style White Bean Burger with Fried Egg and
Avocado
Serves: 1
Preparation time: 5 minutes
Cooking time: 20 minutes

Ingredients:

1 cup (250ml) white Kidney Beans, drained and mashed
8oz (230g) Portobello mushrooms, grilled and finely
chopped
½ cup (125ml) Spelt flakes
½ cup (125ml) marinated Artichoke Hearts, chopped and
patted dry
2 Tbsp (30ml) sun-dried Tomatoes, finely chopped
1 tsp (5ml) balsamic vinegar
4 cups (1ℓ) Mixed Greens
Garnish
4 eggs, fried sunny side up
½ Avocado, sliced
¼ tsp (1ml) sea salt and pepper

Method:

Preheat oven to 400 F (200 C)
Line a baking sheet with parchment paper and set aside.
Using clean hands, combine the first 6 ingredients and
form into 4 equal-sized patties. Place onto lined baking
sheet and bake for 20-minutes.

Divide greens equally between 4 plates. Remove patties
from oven and place over the bed of greens. Garnish each
burger with a fried egg (if desired). Divide avocado slices
evenly between burgers and sprinkle each evenly with
sea salt and pepper.

Macronutrients:

Protein: 14g
Carbs: 24 g
Fats: 3g

Calories: 281

Couscous Salad with Tuna and Avocado

Serves: 1
Preparation time: 10 minutes
Cooking time: 30 minutes

Ingredients:

70g Couscous
125g Kidney Beans
250g Cherry Tomatoes
150g Spinach
1 Pepper
60g of light Feta
150g Tuna
½ Onion
100g Avocado

Method:

Cook the Couscous and let it cool.
Combine everything except avocado and feta and mix thoroughly.
Top with avocado and feta.
Season with lemon pepper/garlic/fresh lemon/balsamic

Macronutrients:

Protein: 76g
Carbs: 97g
Fat: 24g

Calories: 884

Herb Garden Beef Burger

Serves: 4

Preparation time: 10 minutes

Cooking time: 15 minutes

Ingredients:

1 cup (250ml) chopped fresh Herb Mix (dill, basil, parsley, mint and rosemary), divided

1lb (450g) extra-lean Ground Beef

2 tsp (10ml) ground Cumin

¼ tsp (1ml) each Sea Salt and Pepper

Sauce

½ cup (125ml) Low-Fat plain Greek yogurt

1 tsp (5ml) minced/crushed Garlic

½ tsp (2,5ml) Lime Zest

Method:

Measure out 2 Tbsp (30ml) of herb mixture and set aside. Using clean hands, combine remaining herbs, beef, cumin, salt and pepper, and form into 4-equal sized patties.

Grill at med-high heat for 5 to 7 minutes per side, or until cooked as desired.

Stir together reserved 2 Tbsp of herbs (30ml), yogurt, garlic and lime zest. Divide yogurt mixture evenly between burgers.

Macronutrients (per burger):

Protein: 32g
Carbs: 3g
Fat: 10g

Calories: 234

Beef and Rice Mash

Serves: 2
Preparation time: 5 minutes
Cooking time: 5 minutes

Ingredients:

16oz (450g) lean, Ground Beef
1 cup (250ml) cooked Rice
1 Swanson Beef flavor pack
1 Tbsp (15ml) dry Parsley
2 Tbsp (30ml) Fat Free Chicken Broth (in the box)
¼ cup (63ml) Water
1 Tbsp (15ml) Garlic Powder
Season-All to taste (about 2 Tbsp)

Method:

Put the ground beef (mince) in a deeper non-stick pan with a lid and add season-all, garlic powder, and dry parsley and begin to brown on medium heat. As soon as meat begins to brown, stir and then add the cooked rice, flavor packet, water, and broth. Cover and allow to simmer for 15 minutes, stirring 3-4 times.

Macronutrients (per serve):

Protein: 96g
Carbs: 246g
Fat: 32g

Calories: 894

Avocado Lime Chicken

Serves: 1
Preparation time: 5 minutes
Cooking time: 5 minutes

Ingredients:

¼ cup (63ml) Brown Rice
6 oz. (170g) grilled Chicken
½ Lime
1 Avocado
¼-½ packet Stevia

Method:

Grill the chicken breast.
Boil/steam the brown rice.
Cut the Avocado into small cubes while the chicken and
rice cooks.
Squeeze the juice from the lime and add 1/4-1/2 packet
of stevia.
Place the rice, chicken, and avocado into a
bowl/tupperware. Pour the lime juice on top. Mix it all
together. You can add cilantro or whatever you want to it
after that.

Macronutrients:

Protein: 54g
Carbs: 45 g
Fat: 37g

Calories: 726

Marinated Chicken Enchiladas
Servings: 6
Preparation time: 15 minutes
Cooking time: 35 minutes
Basting time: Overnight

Ingredients:
1lb. (450g) boneless, skinless Chicken Breasts, cut into cubes
1 tsp (5ml) Olive Oil
Juice of 1 Lime
1 tsp (5ml) Chili Powder
2 Scallions, minced
Salt and Pepper to taste
1 (15-oz.) can Black Beans, drained and rinsed
6 (6-inch/15cm) Whole-Wheat Tortillas
2/3 cup (180ml) Reduced-Fat shredded Mexican cheese blend or Monterey Jack cheese, divided
1½ cups (375ml) canned Enchilada Sauce

Method:

In a medium bowl, combine the chicken with the olive oil, lime juice, chili powder, scallions, salt, and pepper.
Cover and marinate in the refrigerator for at least 1 hour and up to 24 hours.
Preheat the oven to 375°F (190°C)
Remove the chicken from the marinade and discard the excess.
Heat the olive oil in a nonstick skillet over medium heat. Add the chicken and sauté for 7 to 8 minutes until chicken is cooked through. Remove the chicken to a bowl and add the black beans.
Divide the chicken-and-bean filling among six tortillas. Top each with 1 Tbsp. of the cheese. Roll up each tortilla and place seam-side down in a baking dish coated with cooking spray. Pour the sauce over the enchiladas and bake, covered, for about 20 minutes.
Add the remaining cheese and bake, uncovered, for 5 minutes until cheese melts.

Macronutrients (per serve):
Protein: 26g
Carbs: 30g
Fat:9g

Calories 305

Spanish Rice

Serves: 8
Preparation time: 10 minutes
Cooking time: 30 minutes

Ingredients:

1lb (450g) lean Ground Turkey

1-15oz can Tomato Sauce

1-14.5oz can Diced Tomatoes

1 11oz Diced Tomatoes with Chili Peppers

2 cups (500ml) uncooked instant Brown Rice

1 cup (250ml) Water

2½ tsp (12,5ml) Chili Powder

2 tsp Worcestershire sauce

Method:

Brown turkey in skillet, drain off fat and discard.

Return drained turkey to skillet. Add tomato sauce, tomatoes, rice water, chili powder and Worcestershire sauce. Stir to mix ingredients. Cover and simmer 20 to 25 minutes. Stir before serving.

Macronutrients (per serve):

Protein: 18g

Carbs: 44g

Fat:7g

Calories 310

Asian Flank Steak and Stir-Fry

Serves: 6

Preparation time: 30 minutes

Cooking time: 20 minutes

Ingredients:

4 Tbsp (60ml) Light Soy Sauce, divided

1 Tbsp (15ml) Rice Vinegar

1½ Tbsp (22.5ml) Arrowroot or Cornstarch, divided

1lb (450g) flank Steak, trimmed of all fat

¾ cup (180ml) Low-Fat, reduced-sodium Beef or Bhicken Broth, divided

4 Tbsp (20ml) Hoisin Sauce

1 tsp (5ml) Chili Puree with Garlic

1 Tbsp (15ml) Canola Oil, divided

3 cloves Garlic, minced

1 Tbsp (15ml) minced Ginger

2 stalks Celery, sliced

2 cups (500ml) sliced Broccoli

1 medium Red Pepper, cut into strips

1½ (375ml) cups Snow Peas

Method:

In a bowl, combine 2 Tbsp. soy sauce, rice vinegar, and ½ Tbsp. of the arrowroot or cornstarch.

Add steak to the mixture and let marinate for 15 minutes. In another bowl, combine ½ cup broth with remaining soy sauce, remaining arrowroot or cornstarch, Hoisin sauce, and chili puree; set aside.

Heat half the oil in a wok or skillet. Add the beef and marinade; stir-fry for 3 minutes. Remove the beef and set aside in a bowl.

Heat remaining oil. Add the garlic and ginger, and stir-fry for 30 seconds.

Add the celery, broccoli, and red pepper. Add the remaining broth. Cover. Steam 2 to 3 minutes.

Add the snow peas and cook 1 to 2 minutes more. The vegetables should be crisp.

Add in the sauce and cook 1 minute.

Add in the beef and serve.

Macronutrients (per serve):

Protein: 19g
Carbs: 12g
Fat:7g

Calories 185

Protein Pumpkin Pie

Serves: 1
Preparation time: 5 minutes
Cooking time: 45 minutes
Chilling Time: 5 hours

Ingredients:

½ cup (125ml) canned Pumpkin or Butternut Squash
6oz (175ml) non-fat Greek Yogurt
1 egg
1 Tbsp (15ml) Protein Powder
Cinnamon or Pumpkin Pie Spice to taste.

Method:

Pre-heat oven to 375°F (190°C).
Spray a medium-sized round with non-stick spray.

Mix all the ingredients together and pour into baking dish.
Bake for 45 minutes.
Refrigerate overnight or 4-5 hours.

Macronutrients:

Protein: 31g
Carbs: 19g
Fat: 5g

Calories: 245

Baked Chicken

Serves: 6
Preparation time: 5 minutes
Cooking time: 20 minutes

Ingredients:

6 large boneless skinless Chicken Breasts
1½ cups (375ml) Chicken Broth
¾ tsp (4ml) Onion Powder
¾ tsp (4ml) Garlic Salt
Fresh Ground Black Pepper to taste

Method:

Preheat oven to 350°F (180°C)
Rinse, and pat chicken breasts dry.
Spray a small, shallow baking dish with cooking spray.
Sprinkle chicken with onion powder, garlic salt, and pepper.
Place in baking dish.
Add chicken broth to dish.
Bake 20 minutes or until no longer pink.

Macronutrients (per serve):

Protein: 25.4g
Carbs: 0.7g
Fat: 3.2g

Calories 141.3

Turkey Power Balls

Serves: 6 (2 power balls per serve)
Preparation time: 10 minutes
Cooking time: 25 minutes

Ingredients:

40oz (1.13Kg) Lean Ground Turkey
2 large Eggs Whites
6 Portobello Mushrooms
Dill Weed
Seasoned Italian Herbs
2 slices of Monterey Jack cheese
Black Pepper
A pinch of Sea Salt

Method:

Pre-heat the oven to 320°F (110°C)
Peel and dice the Portobello mushrooms and add into a
large mixing bowl
Add the ground turkey into the bowl along with a
tablespoon each of Dill Weed and Italian Herbs. Add a ½
teaspoon of black pepper and a pinch of sea salt.
Crack the eggs and separate the whites from the yolk.
Add the whites into the bowl.
Mix everything with your hands, ensuring that there is
even distribution of all ingredients throughout the
mixture.
Once mixed, tear small pieces of the Monterey Jack
cheese and add it in evenly to the mix.
Spray a baking tray with non-stick spray
Roll the mixture into 12 golf-sized balls and place on tray.

Place in oven and leave for approximately 18-22 minutes until slightly browned.

Macronutrients (per serve):

Protein: 47g
Carbs: 0g
Fat: 5.4g

Calories 230

Honey Nut Barbeque Chicken Fingers

Serves: 2
Preparation time: 10 minutes
Cooking time: 15 minutes

Ingredients:

6 skinless Chicken Breast tenders
½ cup (125ml) Fiber One Honey Clusters, crushed
½ cup (125ml) ground Honey Roasted Almonds
2 Egg Whites, slightly beaten
1 tsp organic barbecue sauce
Pepper to taste
Finely chopped garlic to taste

Method:

Preheat the oven to 450°F (220°C)

In a shallow dish, combine the egg whites and barbecue sauce.
In another dish mix the crushed cereal, ground almonds,

garlic and pepper.

Dip the chicken pieces into the egg dish, and then coat with the crumb mixture.

Bake about 12 minutes or until the chicken is fully cooked.

Macronutrients (per serve):

Protein: 35g
Carbs: 14g
Fat: 12g

Calories: 300

Chicken Egg White Pizza

Serves: 1
Preparation time: 5 minutes
Cooking time: 5 minutes

Ingredients:

4oz (115g) Boneless Skinless Chicken Breasts
4 large Egg Whites
¼ cup (63ml) Tomato Sauce
1 cup, (250ml) chopped Peppers, Sweet, Green
2 Tbsp (30ml) Peppers, Sweet, Red
2 Tbsp (30ml)Mexican Style Four Cheese
2 Tbsp (30ml) Onions

Method:

On Medium heat thoroughly cook egg whites in small round pan.
Season with pepper, garlic or any other "pizza-y" seasoning you like.
flip egg whites over and add 1/4 cup tomato sauce, chopped vegetables, grilled chicken and cheese.
Reduce heat to medium low and cook until the cheese is melted on top.
Serve.

Macronutrients:

Protein: 47.4g
Carbs: 17.2g
Fat: 10.8g

Calories: 342

Curry Rice

Serves: 2
Preparation time: 10 minutes
Cooking time: 20 minutes

Ingredients:|

2 cups (500ml) cooked Rice, preferably pre-cooked and refrigerated
200g diced Chicken Breast
100g mixed Frozen Vegetables (substitute with fresh if you prefer)
2 Whole Eggs
1 tsp (5ml) Curry Powder
2 cloves Garlic
5g Ginger
1 Tbsp (15ml) Soy Sauce
1 Tbsp (15ml) Oyster Sauce

Method:

Marinate diced chicken breast in half of the soy sauce and oyster sauce
Fry chicken breast over high heat until cooked. Set this aside
Beat eggs, and make very thin omelets, (makes 3-4 thin omelets). Set these aside after slicing
Add a dash of oil to a hot wok and cook finely chopped garlic cloves + ginger for a few seconds
add pre-cooked rice to the pan
Immediately add curry powder and remaining soy sauce and oyster sauce.

Mix into rice

Add mixed frozen vegetables, omelet and chicken, cook for a couple of minutes then serve

Macronutrients (per serve):

Protein: 36g
Carbs: 82g
Fat: 8g

Salmon Balls

Serves: 5
Preparation time: 5 minutes
Cooking time: 5 minutes

Ingredients:

150g Salmon
80-120g Cottage Cheese
20-35g Breadcrumbs

Method:

Preheat oven to 350°F (180°C)

Put the salmon and cottage cheese in a bowl and mix well.
Roll the salmon in some breadcrumbs and ensure they are well covered.

Bake for 20minutes.
Makes roughly 5 balls.

Macronutrients (per serve):

Protein: 55.1g
Carbs: 17.9g
Fat: 10.2g

Calories: 356

Peanut Butter Chicken
Serves: 1
Preparation time: 70 minutes
Cooking time: 25 minutes

Ingredients:

8oz (230g) Chicken
1 Tbsp (15ml) Peanut Butter
1½ Tbsp (22.5ml) Soy Sauce
Ginger
Garlic powder
Hot sauce
Cayenne pepper (optional)

Method:

Preheat oven to 450°F (220°C)

Mix everything in together except for peanut butter, and
let marinate for at least an hour. Place on foil, spread the
peanut butter over the chicken.
Cover and bake for 22-25 minutes.

Open and broil for 1 minute.

Macronutrients

Protein: 54g
Carbs: 6g
Fat: 19g

Calories: 440

Baked Pineapple Chicken

Serves: 8
Preparation time: 5 hours
Cooking time: 45 minutes

Ingredients:

3lb (1.4kg) Chicken Breast

20oz (567g) Unsweetened Pineapple Chunks

2 Tbsp (30ml) Sugar Free Syrup

2 Tbsp (30ml) Reduced Sodium Soy Sauce

¼ tsp (2ml) Black Pepper

½ Sweet Onion (around 150g)

½ tsp (2ml) Ground Ginger

1 tsp (5ml) Pure Lemon Juice

3-4 Slices of a Naval Orange

Method:

Chop your onion. Cut your naval orange slices in half.
Combine all of your ingredients together aside from the
chicken into a bowl. Mix them together. Add your chicken
and mix into a large ziploc bag.

Remove air from bag and mix everything together once
the bag is sealed.

Let marinate in the fridge for at least 2-5 hours (overnight
works even better).

Preheat oven to 375°F (190°C)

Remove and place into a baking dish. Bake for 45
minutes.
Serve hot.

Macronutrients (per serve):

Protein: 47.25g
Carbs: 11.37g
Fat: 1.37g

Calories: 247

Slow Cooked Chicken Stew
Serves: 10
Preparation time: 15 minutes
Cooking time: 5 hours

Ingredients:

4lb (1.8Kg) Chicken Breast
1 Red Onion, chopped
1 Can (10.75 Ounces/305g) 98% Fat Free Cream of
Mushroom Soup
½ tsp (2.5ml) Lemon & Pepper
1½ tsp (7.5ml) Minced Garlic (or 3 Cloves)
1 tsp (5ml) Italian Seasoning
6oz (170g) Mushrooms
2 Large Sweet Potatoes
2 Russet Potatoes
12oz(340g) Carrots
2 Cups (500ml) Water
1 Packet (24g) Onion Gravy Mix

Method:

Chop up your Red Onion, Sweet Potatoes, Russet
Potatoes, Carrots, and Mushrooms.
Cut your Chicken Breasts into 1 inch pieces.

Combine all of your ingredients into the slow cooker.
Cook on high for 4-5 hours.
Serve.

Macronutrients (per serve):

Protein: 45.6g
Carbs: 36g
Fat: 3.3g

Calories: 356

Italian Slow Cooked Chicken

Serves: 12
Preparation time: 15 minutes
Cooking time: 8 hours

Ingredients:

4 ½lb (2Kg) Chicken Breast meat
½ tsp (2.5ml) Black Pepper
1 tsp (5ml) Mrs. Dash Italian Medley (or Italian Seasoning)
½ Red Onion, chopped
2 tsp Minced Garlic (4 Cloves)
1 pct (20g) Dry Italian Salad Dressing Mix
1 can (10.5oz / 298g) 98% Fat Free Cream of Mushroom
½ cup (125ml) Water
8oz (240g) Fat Free Cream Cheese
1½ cups (375ml) Baby Bella Mushrooms (around 100g)

Method:

Chop chicken breasts into halves.
Combine all of the ingredients into slow cooker. Stir

ingredients together until mixed.

Cook on low for 6-8 hours stirring after 3-4 hours.

Macronutrients (per serve):

Protein: 50g
Carbs: 6g
Fat: 1.75g

Calories: 308

Sloppy Joes
Serves: 7
Preparation time: 10 minutes
Cooking time: 25 minutes

Ingredients:

1 Green Pepper, chopped
1 Red Pepper, chopped
1 Sweet Onion, chopped
2 Carrots, chopped.
1 Tbsp (15ml) Olive Oil
2lb (900g) Lean Ground Beef
1 tsp (5ml) Minced Garlic (or 2 Cloves)
8oz (227g) No Salt Added Tomato Sauce
10 Tbsp (150ml) Hickey & Brown Sugar BBQ Sauce
5 tsp (25ml) Sriracha
1 Tbsp (15ml) Worcestershire sauce

Method:

Heat a skillet over a medium flame and add olive oil.
Add the Green Pepper, Red Pepper, and Sweet Onion, and fry for approximately 3 minutes.

Once cooked add your lean ground beef and brown.

After your beef has browned reduce the burner to low, and add in the rest of your ingredients.
Mix everything together.
Let it simmer on low heat for around 10-15 minutes.
Once your sauce starts to thicken up, it's done

Macronutrients (per serve):

Protein: 26.3g
Carbs: 31.6g
Fat: 6.6g

Calories: 251

Creamy Artichoke Chicken

Serves: 2
Preparation time: 10 minutes
Cooking time: 20 minutes

Ingredients:

2 Skinless Chicken Breast
½ cup (125ml) Zoi Greek Yogurt Nonfat Plain Greek
Yogurt
6 tsp (30ml) Dijon Mustard
1 cup (250ml) flowerets Broccoli Flower Clusters
½ cup (125ml) Trader Joe's Artichoke Hearts

Method:

Preheat your oven to 350 F (180 C)

Grind the broccoli in a food processor, mix with artichoke
hearts, Greek yogurt, and dijon mustard.
Coat top of chicken breasts with the mix. Place in a
shallow oven-proof dish.
Bake for 15-20 minutes.

 Macronutrients (per serve):

Protein: 38g
Carbs: 16g
Fat: 2g

Calories 242

Spicy Coconut Chicken Tenders

Serves: 2
Preparation time: 10 minutes
Cooking time: 25 minutes

Ingredients:

2 tsp (10ml) Sriracha Hot Chili Sauce
4 oz (135g) Chicken Breast Tenderloins
4 Tbsp (60ml) raw Unsweetened Shredded Coconut
2 Tbsp (30ml) All Whites 100% Liquid Egg Whites
12 oz (355g) Chicken Breast

Method:

Preheat the oven to 350F(180 C)
Place the shredded coconut on a plate and spread it out some.
Mix the liquid egg whites and sriracha together.
Dip the raw chicken in this mix. Then roll the tenders on a plate that has the coconut shreds on it. Repeat this process and make certain the chicken tenders are well covered.
Spray a baking tray with non-stick spray, ensure that it is well covered.
Place the chicken on the baking sheet and bake for 25 minutes.

Recommended Toppings:

Sriracha
Cinnamon

Macronutrients (per serve):

Protein: 26g
Carbs: 7g
Fat: 13g

Calories: 260

Peanut Butter Chicken

Serves: 1
Preparation time: 5 minutes
Cooking time: 5 minutes

Ingredients:

5oz (150 g) Chicken Breast
½ Onion, medium, chopped
100 ml Almond Milk
20 g Peanut Butter
1 clove Garlic
¼ Hot Chili Pepper
1 tsp (5ml) Ginger
1 packet Sweeteners (Splenda, Sucralose)

Method:

Fry onion and chicken breast on a medium heat until just cooked
While chicken an onion is cooking, mix up all other ingredients in a blender
When chicken is just cooked, add your sauce into the hot pan and bring to a boil, simmering to desired consistency

Macronutrients:

Protein: 50g
Carbs: 14g
Fat: 23g

Calories: 467

Chicken Avocado Burger Patties
Serves: 4
Preparation time: 5 minutes
Cooking time: 5 minutes

Ingredients:

½ cup (125ml) Cilantro
1 Tbsp (15ml) Onion Powder
¼ tsp (1ml) Black Pepper
1 Avocado
1 Tbsp (15ml) Lime Juice
½ cup (125ml) chopped Scallions or Spring Onions
2¼ cups (560ml) Extra Lean Ground Chicken
¼ tsp (1ml) Sea Salt
2 tsp (10ml) Minced Garlic
1 tsp (5ml) Garlic & Herb Seasoning Blend
¼ cup (63ml) Whole Wheat Bread Crumbs

Method:

Preheat oven to 350 F (180 C)

In a large mixing bowl combine all the ingredients together.
Use hands to mix ingredients, turning and mixing

thoroughly.

Form 4 med sized patties with hands and put on baking sheet.

Cook on one side for 18-20 min, flip and cook other side for same amount.

Serve and enjoy.

Macronutrients (per serve):

Protein: 27g
Carbs: 13g
Fat: 16g

Calories: 302

Tuna Melt

Serves: 1
Preparation time: 5 minutes
Cooking time: 5 minutes

Ingredients:

½ can (6.5 oz), Tuna chunks in Water, drained
2 slices Arnold Low Carb Multi Grain Bread
1 Tbsp (15ml) Fat Free Mayonnaise
2 slices Borden Fat Free Single Cheese Slices
A pinch Morton Sea Salt
Dash Black Pepper
1 tsp (5ml) Texas Pete Hot Sauce

Method:

Mix all ingredients together in a bowl except the cheese and bread.
Place cheese on bread and mixture followed by other bread slice and toast until cheese has melted.

Serve hot.

Macronutrients:

Protein: 40g
Carbs: 27g
Fat: 5g

Calories: 290

Chicken Pot Pie

Serves: 10
Preparation time: 15 minutes
Cooking time: 6 hours

Ingredients:

5lb (2.25Kg) Chicken Breast
3 Cans (32.25 Ounces/915g) Healthy Request/Fat Free Cream of Chicken Soup
1 Can (10 3/4 Ounces/305g) 98% Fat Free Cream of Celery
1 Can (10 3/4 Ounces/305g) 98% Fat Free Cream of Mushroom
1½ tsp (7.5ml) Black Pepper
1 tsp (5ml) Garlic Salt
1 tsp (5ml) Onion Powder
5 Packets/Cubes Low/No Sodium Chicken Bouillon
1½ cups (375ml) Sliced Mushrooms
1 cup (250ml) Chopped Celery
1 cup (250ml) Chopped Carrots
16oz (470ml) Frozen Mixed Vegetables
8 Medium Red Potatoes

Method:

Chop up Celery, Carrots, and Red Potatoes.
Cut your Chicken Breasts in half. Combine all of your ingredients into the slow cooker.
Mix everything together.
Cook on high for 5-6 hours.

Macronutrients (per serve):

Protein: 69g
Carbs: 43.9g
Fat: 4.7g

Calories: 494

Spicy Chicken Lentils
Servings: 8
Preparation time: 10 minutes
Cooking time: 6 hours

Ingredients:

3½lb (1.57kg) Chicken Breasts
1½ Tbsp (22.5ml) Olive Oil
1½ tsp (7.5ml) Minced Garlic (or 3 Cloves)
1 Sweet Onion
6oz (170g) Carrots
1 tsp (5ml) Basil
1½ cups (375ml) Lentils
4 tbsp (60ml) Sriracha
1 cup (250ml) BBQ Sauce
2 cups (500ml) Water

Method:

Take out your chicken breasts, trim off the fat , and cut
into halves.
Chop up your sweet onion and carrots.
Combine everything into your slow cooker.
Cook on low for 6 hours.

Macronutrients (per serve):

Protein: 63g
Carbs: 39.75g
Fat: 4.13g

Calories: 448

Spicy Turkey Chili

Serves: 1
Preparation time: 7 minutes
Cooking time: 10 minutes

Ingredients:

4oz (120g) Extra-lean Ground Turkey
¾ cup (180ml) Black Beans
½ cup (125ml) Corn (steamed)
1 packet McCormick's Chili
⅓ cup (83ml) Tomato Paste
⅓ cup (83ml) diced Tomatoes
¼ cup (63ml) chopped Fresh Basil (optional)
1 Jalapeno Pepper (diced, optional)
Seasonings to taste:
½ Tbsp (7.5ml) each Paprika, Cumin, Cayenne, Pepper
Cheese (optional): 1 oz (30g) Goat, Feta, or Low-fat
Mozzarella Cheese

Method:

Season ground turkey with paprika, cumin, cayenne, and
pepper.
Set a skillet on medium heat and lightly spray with
coconut oil. Add meat.

Chop the meat as it cooks in the skillet using a spatula. When the meat is nearly cooked, add in the chili seasoning and tomato paste. Stir.

Add black beans (with some juice), corn, basil, and any other vegetables.

Reduce the skillet to low heat and cover. Let it simmer and cook for 8-10 minutes.

Remove the skillet from the heat and let it cool. Top with cheese if desired.

Macronutrients:

Protein: 46g
Carbs: 50g
Fat: 3g

Calories 395

Serves: 1

Preparation time: 10 minutes

Cooking time: 25 minutes

Ingredients:

4oz (120g) cooked rotisserie Chicken (pulled)

⅓ cup (83ml) Whole Wheat or Durum Wheat Pasta Shells

½ up (125ml) Chicken Broth

1 Tbsp (15ml) 2% Greek Yogurt

¼ cup (63ml) diced Carrots

¼ cup (63ml) chopped Celery

¼ cup (63ml) diced Mushrooms (optional)

Fresh parsley

Seasonings to taste:

1 tsp (5ml) each cumin, pepper, garlic, onion powder,

Mrs. Dash poultry seasoning

Method:

Preheat oven to 405 F (210 C).

In a pot, boil and cook your wheat pasta. Rinse and set aside.

Dice your raw carrots and mushrooms.

Weigh and separate 4 oz baked chicken meat. In a small disposable ramekin or baking dish, add chicken, pasta, Greek yogurt, veggies, and seasonings. Stir with a spoon or mini-spatula.

Pour chicken broth over the mixture. Ensure that a majority of the noodles are covered so that they won't burn when baking.

Top with fresh parsley.

Bake in the oven for 20-25 minutes. Remove from the oven and enjoy.

Macronutrients:

Protein: 39g
Carbs: 33g
Fat: 3g

Calories 347

Teriyaki Salmon
Servings: 3
Preparation time: 60 minutes
Cooking time: 10 minutes

Ingredients:

2 Tbsp (30ml) Olive Oil
3 Tbsp (45ml) Soy Sauce
3 Tbsp (45ml) Sugar-Free Ketchup
2 Tbsp (30ml) Onion Soup Mix Powder
1 Tbsp (15ml) Splenda
½ tsp (2.5ml) minced Garlic
¼ tsp (1ml) Onion Powder
Three 6-oz. (360g) Salmon Steaks

Method:

Combine olive oil, soy sauce, sugar-free ketchup, onion soup mix powder, and Splenda in a bag.
Place salmon filets in the bag and then let sit for about an hour to marinate.
Remove filets from bag and place on the grill for 4-5

minutes per side.

Serve with freshly-steamed vegetables and quinoa or brown rice.

Macronutrients (per serve):

Protein: 46.6g
Carbs: 5.9g
Fat: 7g

Calories: 363

Field of Greens

Serves: 1
Preparation time: 5 minutes
Cooking time: 5 minutes

Ingredients:

8oz (160g) pasture raised Veal
Sea salt
Chives
Ghee
3 cups Romaine lettuce
1 Tbsp (15ml) Macadamia Nut oil
1 tsp (5ml) Balsamic Vinegar

Method:

Heat ghee in skillet to coat the pan. Insert veal. Season with salt and chives.

Brown meat and flip a few times it cooks pretty quick on medium heat for about 10 minutes.

Toss romaine with oil and vinegar; serve immediately.

Macronutrients:

Protein: 51g
Carbs: 8g
Fat: 2g

Calories: 296

Lobster Boat
Serves: 1
Preparation time: 5 minutes
Cooking time: None

Ingredients:

6-8oz (170g) Lobster (ideally claw meat)
1 Tbsp (15ml) light Mayonnaise
Juice from 1/4 Lemon
¼ Bell Pepper, diced
¼ Onion, diced
1 stalk Celery, diced
3-4 Romaine Lettuce heart leaves
Salt and Pepper and other spices, to taste

Method:

Remove lobster meat from shell and cut or tear into
chunks. Place in a bowl.
Add diced vegetables to the lobster then mix in the mayo,
lemon juice, and spices.
Fill the Romaine heart leaves with lobster salad.
Serve

Macronutrients:

Protein: 42g
Carbs: 8g
Fat: 6g

Calories: 260

Spicy Turkey Meatballs
Serves: 4
Preparation time: 10 minutes
Cooking time: 20 minutes

Ingredients:

1½lb (675g) ground Turkey
1 large Egg
2 large Egg whites
¾ cup (180ml) Oats
2 Tbsp. (30ml) minced Jalapeno Pepper
½ tsp (2.5ml) Chili Pepper
¼ cup (63ml) Salsa
½ finely diced green Bell Pepper
½ finely diced red Bell Pepper

Directions:

Preheat oven to 450 F (230 C).
Using your hands, combine all ingredients together in a large bowl.
Form mixture into medium-sized meatballs.
Set meatballs in a baking dish.
Place dish in oven and cook for 12-15 minutes, or until

golden brown.

Top with added salsa.

Macronutrients:

Protein: 19g
Carbs: 7.2g
Fat: 1.7g

Calories: 121

Chicken Cheese Meatballs

Serves: Multiple
Preparation time: 5 minutes
Cooking time: 10 minutes

Ingredients

1½lb (675g) ground Chicken Breast
½ cup (125ml) Low-Fat Mozzarella Cheese
½ cup (125ml) Low-Fat Parmesan Cheese
1 Tbsp (15ml) Oregano
3 Egg Whites
1 cup (250ml) Oats
½ cup (125ml) finely diced Onion

Directions

Preheat oven to 450 F (230 C).
Using your hands, combine all ingredients.
Roll chicken mixture into bite-sized meatballs.
Place meatballs on a greased baking sheet.
Bake for 8-10 minutes or until golden brown.

Macronutrients (per meatball):

Protein: 19.6g
Carbs: 7.2g
Fat: 4.3g

Calories: 155

Chicken Caesar Meatballs
Serves: 10
Preparation time: 10 minutes
Cooking time: 30 minutes

Ingredients

1½lb (675g) ground chicken
3 egg whites
1 cup (250ml) Oats
2 Tbsp (30ml) Low-Fat Caesar salad dressing
½ minced clove Garlic
4 Tbsp (60ml) Low-Fat Parmesan cheese

Directions

Preheat oven 425 F (220 C).
Combine all ingredients in a large bowl.
Roll chicken mixture into about 20 meatballs.
Place each meatball in a muffin cup and bake for 25-28 minutes, or until golden brown.
Once out of the oven, remove from muffin tin.
Before serving, squeeze lemon juice over top.

Macronutrients:

Protein: 19g
Carbs: 7.2g
Fat: 2.8g

Calories: 129

Fish in Foil
Serves: 1
Preparation time: 5 minutes
Cooking time: 20 minutes

Ingredients:

4 oz (120g) Tilapia
Asparagus
½ Lemon, sliced
Juice of ½ a Lemon
Fish seasoning
Pepper

Method:

Preheat oven to375 F (190 C)
Use one piece of foil per fish.
Add lemon juice.
Sprinkle fish seasoning on top.
Add pepper, lemon slices.
Add veggies on top.
Fold into foil down from the top leaving air for steaming
Place each foil on a cookie sheet and bake for 15-20
minutes.

Macronutrients:

Protein: 30g
Carbs: 11g
Fat: 5g

Calories: 209

Chicken Cucumber Salad
Serves: 1
Preparation time: 10 minutes
Cooking time: none

Ingredients:

1 Cucumber
2 stalks of Celery
30g Red Onion
70g Spinach and Kale Greek Yogurt dip
30g Fat-Free Cheddar Cheese
1 can of Chunk Chicken, drained (about 185g)

Directions:

Peel and chop the cucumber, celery, and onion.
Combine all ingredients in a large mixing bowl.
Season to taste
Serve

Macronutrients:

Protein: 51g
Carbs: 19g
Fat: 10g

Calories: 377

Sweet Potato Omelet
Serves: 1
Preparation time: 7 minutes
Cooking time: 10 minutes

Ingredients:
3 large Whole Eggs
1 medium Sweet Potato, baked
3 slices lean Turkey Bacon
¼ (63ml) cup Shredded Cheese
1 Tbsp (15ml) Low-Fat Sour Cream

Method:

Peel sweet potato and mash the flesh. Reheat it in a
skillet or in the microwave.
Cook turkey bacon in a skillet to taste.
Once turkey is done, scramble the eggs and pour them
into a non-stick skillet set to medium heat. Cover the
entire skillet surface in a thin layer of egg. Let the eggs set
and then carefully flip it over.
Spread sweet potato on one side of the eggs.
Sprinkle cheese on top of sweet potato.
Place bacon on top of cheese and sweet potato.

Spread sour cream on top of bacon.

Fold eggs in half and let sit for a minute or two.

Flip omelet over and let sit for a minute or two.

Remove from heat and place on plate.

Add salt and pepper as desired and enjoy!

Macronutrients:

Protein: 37g
Carbs: 27gg
Fat: 24g

Calories: 485

Thai Spicy Beef Salad

Serves: 1
Preparation time: 10 minutes
Cooking time: 5-10 minutes

Ingredients:

½lb (225g) lean Steak

Salt and pepper, to taste

4 cups (1ℓ) Mixed Greens

2 Tbsp (30ml) each: fresh Mint, Basil, and Cilantro

2 green Onions, sliced

2 Tbsp (30ml) fresh Lime Juice

½ tsp (2.5ml) Lemongrass paste or fresh Lemongrass

1 tsp (5ml) low sodium Soy Sauce

1 tsp (5ml) Chili Flakes

2 tsp (10ml) Fish Sauce

1/2 tsp (2.5ml) Stevia in the Raw

Method:

Season steak with salt and pepper and grill to desired readiness.

In a small bowl, mix greens, mint, basil, and cilantro.

In another small bowl, mix lemongrass, green onions, lime juice, soy sauce, fish sauce, chili flakes, and Stevia.

Slice steak and place on top of greens.

Pour dressing over greens and steak.

Toss lightly and serve.

Macronutrients:

Protein: 36g
Carbs: 18g
Fat: 7g

Calories: 260

Malaysian Curry Prawns

Serves: 4
Preparation time: 10 minutes
Cooking time: 10 minutes

Ingredients:

½lb (225g) large Prawns, with shell/tail
1 Tbsp (15ml) Coconut Oil
1 Tbsp (15ml) fresh Garlic, chopped
1 can light Coconut Milk
1 Tbsp (15ml) Curry Powder
Salt and pepper, to taste

Method:

De-vein the prawns.
Heat coconut oil in large pan over medium high heat and add the garlic.
Rinse prawns and lightly salt and pepper.
Add prawns to pan and sprinkle with curry powder.
Sauté for 2-3 minutes until all prawns are well-seasoned.
Add coconut milk and turn heat to low.
Simmer for 5 minutes.
Serve.

Macronutrients (per serve):

Protein: 15g
Carbs: 4g
Fat: 11g

Calories 172

Chicken Curry
Serves: 2
Preparation time: 7 minutes
Cooking time: 10 minutes

Ingredients:

5oz (150g) boneless Chicken Breast
5 cups (1.25ℓ) sliced raw Mushroom
1 whole Red Pepper
2 cups (250ml) green raw Snap Beans
¼ cup (83ml) canned Chicken Broth
1 cups (250ml) Low-Fat Yogurt
4 tsp (20ml) Cornstarch
4 tsp (20ml) Extra Virgin Olive Oil
2 tsp (10ml) Curry Powder

Method:

Take chicken breasts and cut into medium sized cubes.
Grab a large non-stick deep frying pan and add the
chicken breasts with 1 tablespoon of olive oil. Cook the
chicken in frying pan until its browned and done.
While the chicken is cooking grab another non-stick frying
pan and add mushrooms, pepper, and beans with 2
tablespoons of olive oil. Stir this mixture regularly until its

soft.

Back to the first pan and add chicken broth, yogurt, curry powder, and cornstarch. Stir this mixture regularly until the sauce thickens. Increase heat if needed.

Macronutrients:

Protein: 32g
Carbs: 735g
Fat: 13g

Calories: 373

Beef Chop Suey
Serves: 1
Preparation time: 5 minutes
Cooking time: 15 minutes

Ingredients:

7oz (210g) Beef, fat trimmed.

6 large Egg Whites

1 large Onion, chopped

3 cups (750ml) Danish raw cabbage

2½ stripes Celery

2 cups (500ml) of thin sliced Mushrooms

1½ cups (375ml) mature Soybean

2 cups (500ml) Chinese canned Water Chestnut

2 tsp (10ml) Olive Oil

2 Tbsp (60ml) Apple Cider Vinegar

1 Tbsp (15ml) Soy Sauce

½ cup (125ml) broth bouillon canned, ready to serve beef

Method:

You will need 2 large non-stick frying pans. In the first frying pan add the olive oil and beef and cook until the beef is brown. Don't cook for too long, the beef will go tough and chewy.

While the beef is cooking, in the second frying pan, add 2 tablespoons of olive oil, cabbage, celery, mushrooms, water chestnuts, soybean, vinegar and onion. Cook until entire mixture is hot, and the onions have softened. Now add the soy sauce, beef stock and cooked beef. Cook this mixture for 5-10 minutes.

Macronutrients:

Protein: 50g
Carbs: 38g
Fat: 16g

Calories: 490

Salsa Quinoa Chicken
Serves: 5
Preparation time: 5 minutes
Cooking time: 5 minutes

Ingredients:

2 cups (500ml) Quinoa, uncooked
24oz (720g) cooked Chicken
2 cups (500ml) Salsa
1 cup (250ml) Onion, chopped
Diced Jalapeno to taste (optional)

Method:

Boil quinoa in with 4 cups water. After reaching a raging
boil, turn the heat down to medium-low. Allow quinoa to
cook until only a slight amount of water is left. Pull
quinoa from heat, and let stand covered for 10 minutes.
Extra water will soak into the quinoa.
Mix chicken, salsa and onion in with the quinoa.
Divide evenly into 5 Tupperware containers.

Macronutrients:

Protein: 40g
Carbs: 49g
Fat: 6g

Calories: 434

Grilled Tuna Burgers
Serves: 4
Preparation time: 10 minutes
Cooking time: 10 minutes

Ingredients:

450g Tuna
40g Onion, chopped
1 large Carrot, shredded
2 cloves Garlic, finely chopped
4 Egg Whites
20g chopped Chives
40g Bread Crumbs
Spices to taste

Method:

Mix all the ingredients together in a large mixing bowl.
Split ingredients into four patties.
Take a tray and cover with a non-stick piece of baking
paper.
Spray the paper lightly with low fat cooking spray.
Grill patties on both sides until brown.

Serve either with a roll and trimmings, or with rice and vegetables.

Macronutrients:

Protein: 35g
Carbs: 15g
Fat: 1.2g

Calories: 200

Tuna Cheese Melt
Serves: 1
Preparation time: 9 minutes
Cooking time: 6 minutes

Ingredients:

1 5oz (150g) can of Tuna,
2 Tbsp (30ml) of Oatmeal
1 Egg White
Diced Onion to taste
Fresh, minced Garlic to taste
⅓oz (10g) Mozzarella or Cheddar cheese
Salt and Pepper to taste

Method:

Place all ingredients into a mixing bowl.
Mix, or mash ingredients together, and form into a patty.
Place patty into a frying pan, and cook over medium heat.
Cook until slightly brown on both sides.

Macronutrients:

Protein: 26g
Carbs: 4g
Fat: 2g

Calories: 145

Thai Spiced Chicken
Serves: 4
Preparation time: Overnight
Cooking time: 40 minutes

Ingredients:

6 Chicken Breasts cut in half
12oz (350g) natural Non-Fat or Low-Fat Yogurt
2-3 Tbsp (15ml) Thai Red Curry Paste
4 Tbsp (60ml) chopped fresh Cilantro
3 inch (7.5 cm) piece Cucumber
Lime Wedges and Salad Greens to serve

Method:

Preheat your oven to 375 F (190 C).
Put the chicken in a shallow dish in one layer. Blend a
third of the yogurt, the curry paste and three tablespoons
of the cilantro. Season well with salt and pour over the
chicken, turning the pieces until they are evenly coated.
Leave for at least 10 minutes, or in the fridge overnight.

Lift the chicken on to a rack in a roasting tin and roast for
35-40 minutes, until golden.

Blend together the remaining yogurt and cilantro. Finely chop the cucumber and stir into the yogurt mixture. Season. Serve with the chicken and garnish with wedges of lime and salad greens.

Macronutrients (per serve):

Protein: 43g
Carbs: 8g
Fat: 3g

Calories: 166

Snacks & Desserts

Peanut Butter Chocolate Protein Cookies

Chocolate Protein Frozen Yogurt Recipe

Strawberry, Banana and Peanut Butter Ice Cream

Chocolate Orange Protein Balls

Peanut Butter Oatmeal Raisin Muffins

High Protein Chocolate Cake

Rice Pudding

Protein Brownies

Protein Snickers

Peanut Butter Chocolate Cookies

Peanut Butter Ice Cream

Chocolate Mug Cake

Protein Bars

Strawberry and Banana Protein Bar

Banana Bread

Cookies and Cream Rice Krispy Treat

Honey Nut Protein Bars

Peanut Butter Cup Cakes

Protein Oreos

Protein Brownies

High Protein Cheesecake

Chocolate Peanut Butter Protein Bars

Chocolate Peanut Butter Cookie Dough

Protein Pudding

Protein Truffles

Chocolate Cake

Cottage Cheesecake

Amino Acid Jelly

Delicious Dessert Pizza

Chocolate Peanut Butter Wrap

Strawberry Fluff

Banana Flaxseed Muffins

Protein Pancakes/Strawberry Shortcake

Protein Lava Brownie

Protein Mousse Recipe

Protein Cookies and Cream Waffles

Gluten Free Protein Carrot Cake

Boston Cream Donut

Apple Pie Protein Donut

Blueberry Protein Donuts

Chocolate Protein Donuts

Protein Packed Parfait

Coconut-Oat Bars

Cinnamon Scroll

Strawberry Cheesecake

Peanut Butter Chocolate Protein Cookies

Servings: 18
Preparation time: 10 minutes
Cooking time: 2 minutes
Chilling time 1 Hour

Ingredients:

3 cups (750ml) Puffed Brown Rice
1 scoop (30g) Whey Protein Powder (any flavor)
1 cup (250ml) Oats
¼ cup (63ml) Nuts/Dried Fruit
¼ cup (63ml) Stevia
6 tsp (20ml) Dark unsweetened Cocoa
½ cup (125ml) Honey
1 tsp (5ml) Vanilla Extract
¾ cup (180ml) organic Peanut Butter

Method:

Pour 3 cups of brown puffed rice into a mixing bowl.
Add 1 scoop of whey protein
Add 1 cup of whole oats and add some crushed nuts or
dried fruit of your choice

In a microwavable bowl.
Combine Stevia, peanut butter, honey and vanilla extract.
Place in the microwave for 30 second intervals, stirring
frequently, until combined.
Add peanut butter mixture of the crispy rice and stir until
well mixed!
Shape mixture into cookies and place in fridge for an hour

Macronutrients (per serve):

Protein: 5.6g
Carbs: 21.5g
Fat: 7g

Calories: 153

Chocolate Protein Frozen Yogurt
Serves: 1
Preparation time: 5 minutes
Chilling time: 60 minutes

Ingredients:

1 Banana (fresh or frozen)
100g of Full-Fat organic natural live Yogurt
1 Tbsp (15ml) Green & Black's organic Cocoa
40g of Chocolate Protein Powder

Method:

Place the banana, cocoa and protein powder in the
blender and blend until even and crumbly

Add in the yogurt and blend

Pour in to a bowl, jar or dish and freeze for 30-60
minutes.
Test it with your finger on the top to check how far gone
it is.

Macronutrients:

Protein: 41g
Carbs: 31g
Fat: 6g

Calories: 350

Strawberry, Banana and Peanut Butter Ice Cream

Serves: 1
Preparation time: 5 minutes
Cooking time: None

Ingredients:

1 frozen Banana
4 frozen Strawberries
1 Tbsp (15ml) of organic Peanut Butter

Method:

Blend frozen banana on a low speed setting in your blender.

Once banana is well blended, add the 4 frozen strawberries and tablespoon of peanut butter.

Macronutrients:

Protein: 10g
Carbs: 15g
Fat: 10g

Calories: 100

Chocolate Orange Protein Balls
Serves: 1
Preparation time: 5 minutes
Cooking time: 5 minutes

Ingredients:

80g Dates
70g Rolled Oats
50g Peanut Butter
3 scoops (90g) of Chocolate Whey Protein
10g Cocoa
1 Orange
1 sachet powdered Egg Whites
20g shredded Coconut

Method:

Finely grate the rind from your orange and add the rind
along with everything but the coconut in to your blender.
Add in the juice one half of the orange (65ml).

Whizz intermittently until everything comes together in a
soft, balling, sticky fashion.

Put your shredded coconut in to a small bowl. The mix is very sticky, I used a tablespoon to remove around 35g of mixture at a time. Plop one spoonful in to the bowl of coconut and tumble it until covered. You can then remove it and roll it in to a ball with your hands.

Plop, roll and ball 10 times. Try and make them even. I sat my bowl on a scale so I could check how much each blob I removed weighed.

Sit the rolled balls on a plate and fridge them for an hour minimum.

Can then store or eat up as desired!

Macronutrients:

Protein: 10g
Carbs: 14g
Fat: 4g

Calories: 131

Peanut Butter Oatmeal Raisin Muffins

Servings: 8
Preparation time: 10 minutes
Cooking time: 20 minutes

Ingredients:

3g Splenda
1 tsp (5ml) of Baking Powder
10g Peanut Butter powder (PB2)
1 scoop (30g) peanut butter flavored Whey Protein
1 Tbsp (15ml) Greek Yogurt
1 Tbsp (15ml) Regular Yogurt
2 Egg Whites
½ cup (125ml) flavored oatmeal.
10g Complete Pancake Mix

Method:

Crack your Egg Whites and add into a magic bullet, with the yogurts.
Add the dry ingredients, and blend for 2-3 minutes.

Pre-heat Oven to 350 F (180 C)
Ppray a muffin sheet/pan with a nonstick spray
Slowly pour the mixture about half way up the muffin pan.

Bake for 16-20 minutes until a toothpick will come out clean.

Transfer to a cooling rack to cool.

Macronutrients (per serve):

Protein: 5g
Carbs: 6g
Fat:0.5g

Calories: 48

High Protein Chocolate Cake
Servings: 8
Preparation time: 10 minutes
Cooking time:30 minutes

Ingredients:

2 scoops (60g) Chocolate Whey Protein
½ cup (125ml) Whole Wheat Flour
⅓ cup (83ml) unsweetened Cocoa Powder
1 tsp (5ml) Baking Powder
1 tsp (5ml) Baking Soda
1 egg
2 tsp (5ml) Vanilla extract
¼ cup (63ml) Avocado
1 6oz jar baby food fruit + oatmeal mix
Sweetener of choice (splenda/stevia etc.)

Method:

Preheat oven to 350 F (180 C).
Coat baking pan with cooking spray
Mix all dry ingredients in a separate bowl
Slowly add wet mixture into dry ingredient bowl
Blend bowl of ingredients
Bake for 25 minutes

Macronutrients (per serve):

Protein: 8g
Carbs: 14g
Fat:1.8g

Calories: 120

Rice Pudding
Serves: 1
Preparation time: 5 minutes
Cooking time: 5 minutes

Ingredients:

1½ (375ml) cups cooked White Rice
8 oz (230ml) Vanilla Rice Milk
2 Tbsp (30ml) Lactose Free Chocolate or Vanilla Breyer's
Ice Cream

Method:

Place rice in a bullet, or farberware blender, not a regular
blender, add rice milk, and ice cream
Blend till thick, open blender, stir, and add more rice milk
till full
Blend again till creamy/

Macronutrients:

Protein: 35g
Carbs: 78g
Fat:4g

Calories: 490

Protein Brownies
Serves: 9
Preparation time: 15 minutes
Chilling time: 4 minutes

Ingredients:

2 scoops (60g) Vanilla Whey
30g chopped Almonds
3g Cocoa Powder
50g Oats
50ml Almond Milk
30g Roasted Peanuts
3 Tbsp (45ml) crunchy Peanut Butter
Dark chocolate coated thin Rice Cakes for base
90g 60% Dark Chocolate

Method:

Place some rice cakes on an aluminum foil these form the base for the chocolate bites.
Mix all the powders and oats together in a bowl.
Add in the peanut butter and almond milk and stir until you get a thick batter.

Add in the almonds and stir a bit more to mix.

Coat the rice thins with the mixture and spread evenly across the whole base.

Place tray in freezer for 15 minutes until you melt the dark chocolate in a Bain Marie.

Once the dark choc is melted, take the tray out of the freezer. Before pouring the chocolate, place the roasted peanuts on top of the hardened mixture.

Pour the dark chocolate on top and spread evenly with a spatula or spoon.

Place in the fridge for 3-4 hours to get everything firm.

Remove and cut into equal squares.

Macronutrients (per serve):

Protein: 11g
Carbs: 13g
Fat:11g

Calories: 190

Protein Snickers

Serves: 10
Preparation time: 10 minutes
Cooking time: 2 minutes

Ingredients:

Filling
100g Peanut Butter
50g Protein Powder
10g Cocoa
200g Low Fat Greek Yogurt
20g crushed raw Peanuts

Chocolate shell:
80g +85% Chocolate
20g Coconut Oil
Sweetener

Method:

Protein bar:
Mix all ingredients together.
Divide the mixture into 10 equal parts, and shape into a bars

Chocolate cover:
Break the chocolate into small pieces
Melt the coconut oil, (Place container in boiling water,)
Melt the chocolate, add the coconut oil and whisk
Coat the bars with a small amount of chocolate, dip them in the chocolate

Macronutrients (per serve):

Protein: 10.2g
Carbs: 3.5g
Fat: 11.3g

Calories: 156

Peanut Butter Chocolate Cookies

Servings: 8
Preparation time: 5 minutes
Cooking time: 10 minutes

Ingredients:

60g Protein Powder
75ml Almond Milk
3 Tbsp (45ml) of smooth Peanut Butter
15g chopped Almonds
30g Oats
60g Dark Chocolate (60%)

Method:

Preheat oven to 212 F (100 C).
Mix the first 2 ingredients thoroughly. Then add the
peanut butter and continue to blend until smooth.
Mix this paste with the oats and almonds and with a
spoon and stir well.
Fold in the chopped dark chocolate (or chocolate chips).
Form balls out of the mixture and place on cooking tray.
Bake for 5 minutes and then switch off oven and leave for

another 2-3 minutes.

Remove and leave them on the tray to cool.

Macronutrients (per serve):

Protein: 8g
Carbs: 8g
Fat: 7g

Calories 127

Peanut Butter Ice Cream

Serves: 1
Preparation time: 5 minutes
Cooking time: 30 minutes

Ingredients:

100ml Low Fat Milk
3 Tbsp (45ml) of Crispy Peanut Butter
1 scoop (30g) Vanilla Whey Protein

Method:

Mix milk, Peanut Butter and Whey Protein. Heat it in a
pan for 3-4min (until it's creamy).
Place it into the freezer for about 30min.

Macronutrients:

Protein: 38.6g
Carbs: 10.8g
Fat: 22.6g

Calories: 400

Chocolate Mug Cake

Serves: 1
Preparation time: 3 minutes
Cooking time: 1 minutes

Ingredients:

1 Egg White
1 scoop (30g) Chocolate Protein Whey
1 Tbsp (15ml) Cocoa Powder
1 tsp (5ml) Baking Powder
¼ cup (63ml) water or Coconut milk
Non-stick spray

Method:

Mix ingredients in bowl
Spray mug with non stick spray
Pour ingredients into mug and microwave for 40 seconds
Flip over mug and the cake slides out

Macronutrients:

Protein: 30g
Carbs: 6g
Fat: 3g

Calories: 150

Protein Bars

Serves: Multiple
Preparation time: 5 minutes
Cooking time: 15 minutes

Ingredients:

80gr of Oats
2 scoops (60g) of Vanilla or Strawberry Whey Protein
30gr Peanut Butter
20gr Honey
20gr crushed Walnuts
5-10gr Gojie Berries
Enough water to mix all together into a paste.

Method:
Preheat your oven to 300 F (150 C).
Mix everything into a bowl then put into a trey with cooking paper.
Bake for 12 minutes.

Remove and allow to cool slightly, then cut into bars or cubes.

Macronutrients:

Protein 66g
Carbs 90g
Fats 38g

Calories: 920

Strawberry and Banana Protein Bar

Servings: 6
Preparation time: 10 minutes
Cooking time: 35 minutes

Ingredients:

1 cup (280ml) raw Oatmeal
5 scoops (150g) Strawberry Protein Powder
¼ cup (63ml) Fat-Free Cream Cheese
½ cup (125ml) Non-Fat dry Milk Powder
2 Egg Whites
¼ cup (63ml) Water
1½ Bananas, mashed
2 tsp (10ml) Canola oil

Method:

Preheat oven to 330 F (160 C)

Spray a 9x9 square pan with cooking spray & set aside.
In a medium bowl combine oatmeal, Protein powder &
dry milk. Set aside.
In another bowl beat together with an electric hand
mixer, cream cheese, egg whites, bananas, water & oil.
Add the oat mixture & continue to beat until the two are
combined. Pour batter into the prepared pan.
Bake for 30-35 minutes or until toothpick comes out
clean.

Macronutrients (per bar):

Protein 22g
Carbs 22g
Fat 3g

Calories: 203

Banana Bread

Serves: 8
Preparation time: 10 minutes
Cooking time: 50 minutes

Ingredients:

200g almond meal or oatmeal, depending on your carb
requirements
1 cup (250ml) Vanilla Protein Powder
1 tsp (5ml) Baking Powder
1 cup (250ml) Greek Yogurt
4 eggs
½ tsp (2,5ml) salt
2 bananas, mashed

Method:

Preheat your oven to 280 F (140 C).

Mix the eggs and yogurt together
Add in the two mashed bananas.

Once this is nice and smooth, add in the dry ingredients
and mix well.

Pour the mixture into a loaf tin.

Bake for about 50 minutes.

To check to see if it is done, poke a skewer into the middle of the loaf. When it is done, the skewer should come out clean.

Sever cooled

Macronutrients (per serve):

Protein: 24g
Carbs: 12g
Fat: 18g

Calories: 306

Cookies and Cream Rice Krispy Treat

Serves: 1
Preparation time: 10 minutes
Chilling time: 30 minutes

Ingredients:

39g Rice Krispy Cereal
1 scoop (30g) Cookies and Cream Whey Protein
20g Marshmallow Fluff
5g Honey
50g Greek Yogurt

Method:

Combine Dry (Cereal + Whey) in a bowl
Combine Wet (Yogurt, Honey and Fluff) In a small bowl
Take a small square container and coat with cooking
spray and then mix the wet and dry in the larger bowl.
When combined together you will then drop the mixture
into the square container and level off like a square
(Krispy Treat)
Allow to sit in fridge for 20-30 minutes and then enjoy so
it will settle and bind together.

Macronutrients:

Protein: 30g
Carbs: 60g
Fat: 2g

Calories: 380

Honey Nut Protein Bars

Servings: 6
Preparation time: 10 minutes
Chilling time: 1 hour

Ingredients:

120g Oats
2 scoops (60g) High Protein Whey
100g Peanuts
4 Tbsp (10ml) Olive Oil
2 Tbsp (10ml) Honey

Method:

Start by blitzing the peanuts up, add olive oil and continue to blitz until you have peanut butter (1-2 minutes depending on crunchy or smooth).
Mix with all other ingredients in bowl until it starts to combine, add more oil if too dry.
Put mixture in 8x8 baking tray, spread/ pat down until fully spread evenly.
Put it in the fridge to firm up for an hour, take it out and divide into bars. I cut mine into six, store in foil in fridge and enjoy.

Macronutrients:

Protein: 14g
Carbs: 20g
Fat: 3.5g

Calories: 301

Peanut Butter Cup Cakes

Serves: 3
Preparation time: 15 minutes
Freezer time: 2 hours

Ingredients:

118g of powdered Peanut Butter (PB2)
110ml semi-Skimmed Milk
24g Bourneville cocoa
10g Candarel granulated sweetener

Method:

Add water to the PB2 powder to make a paste in a
separate bowl.

Mix the milk, bournville cocoa, and candarel sweetener
together.
Start spooning the PB2 into the mixture until it thickens
up and resembles thick melted chocolate: use only half of
the PB2 mixture, as the other is used for the filling.
Spray 3 cupcake holders with a nonstick spray.
Line the cupcake holders with the chocolate mixture.
Once the cake holders have been lined with the chocolate
mixture, spoon blobs of the leftover PB2 paste into the
cake holders.
Add the rest of the chocolate mixture over the PB2 paste.
Leave it in the freezer for around 2 hours and it hardens
up like regular chocolate.

Macronutrients (per serve):

Protein: 19.6g
Carbs: 22.1g
Fat: 8g

Calories: 206

Protein Oreos
Servings: 7
Preparation time: 10 minutes
Cooking time: 10 minutes

Ingredients:

1 tbsp (15ml) Vanilla Extract
⅓ cup (83ml) Honey
½ scoop (15g) Dymatize Nutrition Elite Casein - Vanilla
¼ cup (63ml) Greek Yogurt
¼ cup (63ml) Almond Meal
1 cup (250ml) Cocoa Powder (Unsweetened)
1 scoop (30g) Chocolate Whey Protein
1 tsp (5ml) Baking Powder
2 tbsp (30ml) Unsweetened Almond Milk
¼ cup (63ml) Unsweetened Applesauce
1 medium Egg
¼ cup (63ml) Lowfat Cottage Cheese

Method:

Preheat oven to 350 F (180 C).

Combine almond meal, cocoa powder, egg, applesauce, vanilla, honey, baking powder and chocolate protein powder.

Form 14 Oreo sized cookies on a greased pan.

Bake for 10 minutes.

For the frosting

Blend cottage cheese, Greek yogurt, 1/2 tbsp of honey, vanilla casein protein and almond milk, when cookies are cooled, place frosting between the cookies.

Macronutrients (per serve):

Protein: 10g

Carbs: 9g

Fat: 5g

Calories: 121

Serves: 1

Preparation time: 3 minutes

Cooking time: 1 minutes

Ingredients:

1 scoop (30g) Chocolate Whey Protein

2 tsp (10ml) of Cocoa Powder

1/4 teaspoon Baking Powder

Method:

Mix together with a little water into a paste and microwave for 1 minute.

Best served with low vanilla fat ice-cream.

Macronutrients:

With 50ml ice-cream:

Protein: 30.4g

Carbs: 38.9g

Fat: 6.7g

Calories: 275

High Protein Cheesecake

Serves: Multiple
Preparation time: 10 minutes
Cooking time: 45 minutes

Ingredients:

3 scoops (90g) High Protein Whey
8oz (230ml) fat free Cream Cheese
6oz (170ml) plain Greek Yogurt
8oz (230ml) Skim Milk
½ cup (125ml) Cottage Cheese
1 egg
½ cup (125ml) Spenda (7 packets)
1 tsp (5ml) Vanilla Extract
2 tsp (10ml) Cinnamon

Method:

Preheat your oven to 350 F (180 C).

Mix everything together
Add some blueberries or strawberries for variation (if
desired)
Bake for 45 minutes

Allow to cool and place in the fridge for a few hours until
cold..
Serve cold

Macronutrients:

Protein: 151g
Carbs 55g
Fat 10g

Calories: 968

Chocolate Peanut Butter Protein Bars
Serves: 6
Preparation time: 10 minutes
Cooking time: 5 minutes

Ingredients:

1½ cups (375ml) Chocolate Whey Protein powder
¾ cup (180ml) Almond Meal
2 Tbsp (30ml) Cocoa powder
¼ cup (63ml) creamy Peanut Butter
½ cup (125ml) milk
100 g Dark Chocolate

Method:

Mix the first 5 ingredients in a bowl until you get a thick paste-like batter. Divide the batter into 6 portions and shape into bars. Chill in the freezer for a few minutes to harden up a bit.

Melt the chocolate slowly over a double boiler. Once melted, add bars one at a time to coat. Stick back in the freezer and enjoy once the chocolate has hardened.

You can also sub in oat or coconut flour for the almond meal, and any other favorite protein powder flavor you like or have on hand

Macronutrients:

Protein: 19g
Carbs 20g
Fat 22g

Calories: 343

Chocolate Peanut Butter Cookie Dough

Serves: 1
Preparation time: 35 minutes
Cooking time: none

Ingredients:

2 tsp (10ml) Peanut Butter
2 scoops (60g) Chocolate Whey Protein
40-50ml Skim Milk

Method:

Mix peanut butter and whey in a bowl and add milk, a little bit at a time, until you have a cookie dough like consistency, put it in the fridge for half an hour and enjoy chocolate peanut butter cookie dough

Macronutrients:

Protein: 56g
Carbs 6g
Fat 19g

Calories: 419

Protein Pudding

Serves: 1
Preparation time: 5 minutes
Cooking time: 5 minutes

Ingredients:

1 cup (250ml) plain Greek Yogurt
1 scoop (30g) Chocolate Whey
3 Tbsp (45ml) unsweetened Cocoa Powder or to taste
Sweetener of choice (optional)

Method:
Stir in the whey and the cocoa powder until completely blended; you should end up with a thick, dark brown paste, add more cocoa if desired.
Serve.

For an added crunch or sweetness, add some nuts, fruit, raw cocoa nibs, etc.
Alternatively, Put it in the freezer for 1-2 hours for a tasty frozen treat.

Macronutrients:

Protein: 52g
Carbs 17g
Fat: 4g

Calories: 330

Protein Truffles

Serves: 10 (3 balls per serve)
Preparation time: 15 minutes
Cooking time: None

Ingredients:

1 cup (250ml) Defatted Peanut Flour
1 cup (250ml) Vanilla Protein Powder
½ cup (12ml) Splenda
⅓ cup (83ml) Torani SF Vanilla Syrup
2 Tbsp (30ml) Butter
2 Tbsp (30ml) Peanut Butter
1 Tbsp (15ml) Vanilla Extract
Cocoa Powder or Chocolate Chips

Method:

Mix all ingredients until a ball is formed. Add more Splenda if too sticky, more syrup if too dry. Roll into 40 balls.
For Buckeyes, melt chocolate chips and drizzle chocolate over refrigerated, formed, dough balls.
For Truffles, roll formed dough balls in cocoa powder. Keep refrigerated.

Macronutrients (per serving):

Protein: 80g
Carbs: 12g
Fat: 3g

Calories: 395

Chocolate Cake

Serves: Multiple
Preparation time: 10 minutes
Cooking time: 35 minutes

Ingredients:

1¾ (430ml) cups All-Purpose Flour
½ cup (125ml) Splenda No Calorie Sweetener, Granulated
½ cup (125ml) Splenda Brown Sugar Blend
¾ cup (180ml) cocoa powder
1½ tsp (7,5ml) baking powder
1½ tsp (7,5ml) baking soda
½ (2,5ml) teaspoon salt
1¼ cups (315ml) low-fat buttermilk
¼ cup (63ml) vegetable oil
2 large eggs, lightly beaten
2 tsp (10ml) vanilla extract
1 cup (250ml) hot strong black coffee

Method:

Preheat oven to 350 F (180 C). Grease a 10 cup bund pan with non-stick cooking spray, set aside.
Blend flour, Splenda Granulated Sweetener, Spenda Brown Sugar Blend, baking powder, baking soda, cocoa powder, protein powder and salt in large mixing bowl.
Combine buttermilk, oil, eggs, vanilla extract, and coffee in a small bowl.
Add flour to mixture, using an electric mixer on medium speed, mix until Smooth (about 2 minutes).
Pour batter into cake pan or bundt pan.

Bake for 30-35 minutes, until an inserted toothpick in center of cake comes out clean. Let cool in pan for 5 minutes.

Macronutrients:

Protein: 36g
Carbs 33g
Fat 70g

Calories: 230

Cottage Cheesecake

Serves: 2
Preparation time: 10 minutes
Cooking time: 24 hours

Ingredients:

600g Cottage Cheese
3 large Egg Whites
1 whole large Egg
10 drops (1ml) Vanilla Flavoring
Cinnamon

Method:

Preheat oven to 320F (160C)

Blend all the ingredients in a food processor
Bake for 20-25 minutes. It should still jiggle slightly if you poke the side. Let it cool in the fridge for 6-24 hours then enjoy.

Macronutrients (per serve):

Protein: 42.5g
Carbs: 13g
Fat: 23g

Calories: 423

Amino Acid Jelly
Serves: 1
Preparation time: 5 minutes
Cooking time: 5 minutes

Ingredients:

2 scoops of Scivation Xtend
1½ Tbsp (22.5ml) gelatin
500ml water (plus 100ml for mixing gelatin)

Instructions:

Mix 2 scoops of Xtend into 500ml of cold water and shake.
Separately mix gelatin into 100ml of hot water. Combine gelatin with Xtend mix and shake well.
Pour into a bowl and place in the fridge. Serve when set!

Makes approx 500grms

Macronutrients:

Protein: 15g (Amino Acids)
Carbs: 0
Fat:0

Calories: 60

Delicious Dessert Pizza

Serves: 4
Preparation time: 10 minutes
Cooking time: 5 minutes

Ingredients:
2¼ Cups (563ml) King Arthur Flour" Whole Wheat Organic
2 cups (500ml) Mixed Berries
¼ cup (63ml) Peaches
½ Banana
¼ tsp (1ml) Sea Salt
1 tsp (5ml) Stevia
1 cup (250ml) warm water
Cinnamon
3 Tbsp (45ml) Chocolate Lean beef Aminos
Vanilla Extract
Pizza Crust Yeast

Method:

Preheat your oven to 425 F (200 C).

Dissolve salt, yeast, and stevia in 1 cup of warm water.
Then mix flour, cinnamon, vanilla extract with the
dissolved salt/yeast/stevia/water mixture. Add the water

in increments until a dough like texture is obtained, Grease a pizza pan.

Wet hands (so dough doesn't stick) spread dough out on pizza pan.
Scatter the Mixed Berries, Peaches, Banana, and Lean beef Aminos over the dough.
Bake for 12 to 15 minutes.

Serve hot

Macronutrients (per serve):

Protein: 15g
Carbs: 42g
Fats: 1.8g

Calories: 334

Chocolate Peanut Butter Wrap

Serves: 1
Preparation time: 5 minutes
Cooking time: None

Ingredients:

1 scoop (30g) Chocolate Protein Powder

1 Tbsp. (15ml) natural Peanut Butter

1 Whole Wheat Wrap

1 Banana

½ packet of Splenda

Method:

Add a bit of water to the protein powder in a bowl and stir until you get the same consistency as peanut butter

Add 1/2 packet of splenda and stir

Spread on whole wheat wrap

Cut up the banana and roll up inside the wrap

Macronutrients:

Protein: 32g

Carbs: 49g

Fats: 10g

Calories 435

Strawberry Fluff

Serves: 1
Preparation time: 5 minutes
Cooking time: None

Ingredients:
½ cup (125ml) or 1DL of Casein-Based Chocolate Protein Powder.
½ cup (125ml)or 1DL of Skimmed Milk.
About 300g of frozen Raspberries.

Method:
Put your protein powder in a bowl.
Pour your milk over the powder and mix it with a spoon
Put your berries in your microwave at low heating power for about five minutes. Be careful not to overdo it and unfreeze them completely because this may mess up your fluff.
When your berries are unfrozen put them in your bowl and mix everything again.
Take out your electronic mixer and mix for about 10 minutes.
The fluff is done when it has grown very big and fluffy.

Macronutrients:

Protein: 33g
Carbs: 30g
Fat: 6g

Calories: 306

Banana Flaxseed Muffins

Serves: 12
Preparation time: 10 minutes
Cooking time: 20 minutes

Ingredients:

½ cup (250ml Flax Seed
3 Bananas, mashed
¼ cup (63ml) Vegetable Oil
½ cup (125ml) Splenda
2 Egg Whites
1½ cups Vanilla Protein Powder
½ tsp (2,5ml) Baking Powder
½ tsp (2,5ml) Baking Soda
¼ cup (63ml) Whole Flax Seeds

Method:

Preheat oven to 350 F (180 C)
In a large mixing bowl, beat together bananas, oil,
Splenda and egg whites.
Mix in the remaining ingredients, folding until smooth.
Lightly grease your muffin pan.
Spoon batter into prepared muffin pan.
Bake for 12-15 minutes or until a toothpick inserted into
a muffin comes out clean.

Macronutrients (per serve):

Protein: 10g
Carbs: 10g
Fats: 3.5g

Calories: 105

Protein Pancakes/Strawberry Shortcake

Serves: 3
Preparation time: 10 minutes
Cooking time: 15 minutes

Ingredients:

2 scoops (60g) Strawberry Whey Protein Powder
¼ cup (63ml) Oats
¾ cup (190ml) Egg Whites
6oz (120g) fresh Strawberries
¼ cup (63ml) Mrs. Butterworth's SF Syrup
50g Reddi-Whip FF Whipped Cream

Method:

Blend the whites, whey, and oats in a blender and put in a cup.
Puree strawberries and syrup in blender, then put in a separate cup.
Heat a skillet to medium heat and coat with some non-stick spray.
Make the pancakes as you normally would. Pour over the strawberry puree and top with whipped cream.

Macronutrients (per serving):

Protein: 23g
Carbs: 17g
Fats: 1g

Calories: 170

Protein Lava Brownie
Serves: 1
Preparation time: 3 minutes
Cooking time: 1 minutes

Ingredients:

2 scoops (60g) Chocolate Protein Powder
2 Tbsp (60ml) Sugar Free Jello Pudding
2 Tbsp (60ml) Sugar Free Maple Syrup
1 Tbsp (15ml) extra Dark Cocoa
2 Egg Whites
2 packets of sweetener (splenda, stevia etc.)

Method:

Place all ingredients into mixing bowl.

Proceed to thoroughly stir, until a thick gooey consistency is achieved.

Microwave for 30 seconds.

Remove and stir.

Microwave for another 30 seconds.

Serve hot.

Macronutrients:

Protein: 60g
Carbs: 10g
Fats: 6g

Calories: 334

Protein Mousse Recipe
Serves: 6
Preparation time: 5 minutes
Cooking time: None

Ingredients:

1 Container (6 Ounces/170g) Plain Fat Free Greek Yogurt
½ Cup (125ml) Pure Pumpkin
½ Banana mashed
½ Tsp (2,5ml) Vanilla Extract
3 Tbsp (45ml) Powdered Peanut Butter
1½ Scoops (45g) Chocolate Protein Powder
2 Tbsp (30ml) Cocoa Powder
3 Packets Sweetener
Mini Graham Cracker Pie Crusts (Optional)

Method:

Combine all of your ingredients together into a bowl or food processor or mixing bowl
Pour your mix into a bowl or on top of your mini graham cracker pie crusts.

Macronutrients (per serve):

Protein: 11.5g
Carbs: 8.1g
Fat: 0.8g

Calories: 86.1

Protein Cookies and Cream Waffles

Serves: 1
Preparation time: 10 minutes
Cooking time: 10 minutes

Ingredients:

1 scoop (30g) Cellucor Cookies and Cream Whey
1 cup (250ml) Liquid Egg Whites
½ cup (125ml) Raw Oats
¼ Cup (63ml) Fiber One Cereal
1 tsp (5ml) Vanilla Extract
1 tsp (5ml) Ground Cinnamon
3 Tbsp (15ml) Unsweetened Baking Coco
Nonstick cooking spray

Method:

Start by heating up the waffle iron at a medium to high heat.
Grind the oats and fiber one cereal in a food processor, and set aside in a separate bowl.
Place the Liquid Egg Whites, and pour them in a blender and add in the fiber one and oat flour. Blend well,
Add the Cookies and Creme whey, baking coco, vanilla extract and blend well.

Spray the waffle iron with a nonstick spray and pour in batter. Sprinkle on the cinnamon (or mix in batter) and press down on the waffle iron. Flip every 2-3 minutes until cooked.

Suggested Toppings:

Peanut Butter
Fat Free Whipped Cream
SF Syrup

Macronutrients: (without toppings):

Protein: 52g
Carbs: 38g
Fat: 6g

Calories: 420

Gluten Free Protein Carrot Cake

Serves: 1
Preparation time: 10 minutes
Cooking time: 45 minutes

Ingredients:

½ cup (125ml) Vanilla Protein Powder
3 Tbsp (35ml) Coconut Flour
½ cup (125ml) gluten-free Oats
1½ cups (375ml) Almond Milk
2 small ripe Bananas, mashed
1 tsp (5ml) Baking Powder
1 (70g) Carrot, grated
1 (70g) Zucchini, grated
2 Tbsp (30ml) Walnuts

Method:

Preheat your oven to 350 F (180 C)

In a medium size mixing bowl combine the protein powder, coconut flour, oats, milk, baking powder, and bananas, and mix well.
With a spoon, mix in the grated carrots, zuchini, and walnuts.

Spray a medium sized bread tin with a nonstick spray and scoop the mixture into it.

Bake for 45 minutes, until cooked. Check by inserting a knife, the blade should be lean on withdrawal. Remove and cool completely before icing.

Mix 1 pack of Quark (250 grams) with 1/8 scoop (16g) of vanilla whey and 1 tsp (5ml) of freshly-shaven vanilla pods (optional).

Macronutrients:

Protein: 26g
Carbs: 22g
Fat: 6g

Calories: 246

Boston Cream Donut

Serves: 4
Preparation time: 15 minutes
Cooking time: 10 minutes

Ingredients:

1 medium Egg, separated
¼ cup (65ml) dry Quaker Old Fashioned Oats
2 large Egg Whites
1 tsp (5ml) Vanilla Extract
¾ tsp (3,5ml) Baking Powder
½ Tbsp (7,5ml) unsweetened Cocoa Powder
¼ tsp (1ml)) Xanthan Gum
1 Tbsp (15ml) Almond Meal Flour
¼ cup (63ml) Lowfat Cottage Cheese
2 tsp (10ml) Almond Milk - Unsweetened Original
½ scoop (20g) Vanilla Whey protein
3 packets Sugar in the Raw or Stevia in The Raw (Packet)
¾ tsp Butter extract

Method:

Preheat your oven to 350 F (180 C).
Grind the oats into a flour. Then add almond flour, vanilla
whey protein, 3 egg whites, baking powder, vanilla
extract, and 1 stevia packet.
Mix well Blend again.
Spray a donut pan with nonstick spray, and scoop batter
into rings.
Bake for 10 minutes.

Topping

Cream, blend the lowfat cottage cheese, egg yolk, 1 stevia packet, 3/4 tsp butter extract, and xanthan gum. Chocolate drizzle, mix the unsweetened cocoa powder, and unsweetened almond milk, and 1 stevia packet. When the donuts are done, remove and top with the icing and chocolate.

Macronutrients (per serving):

Protein: 10g
Carbs: 7g
Fat: 3g

Calories: 94

Apple Pie Protein Donut

Serves: 5
Preparation time: 5 minutes
Cooking time: 5 minutes

Ingredients:

½ cup (125ml) dry Old Fashioned Oats
3 large Egg Whites
1ml Cinnamon
¼ tsp (2ml) Maple Extract
⅓ medium Apple, chopped
½ tsp (2ml) Baking Powder
4 tsp (20ml) Sugar Free Syrup
1 tsp (5ml) Vanilla Extract
¼ scoop (12g) Cellucor Cor-Performance Whey
1 packet Sugar in the Raw or Stevia in The Raw

Method:

Preheat your oven to 350 F (180 C).
Grind oats into a flour. Then add the whey protein, egg whites, baking powder, vanilla extract, maple extract, cinnamon, and 1 stevia packet. Blend again.
Add the chopped apple and swirl it into the batter.
Spray a donut pan with nonstick spray, and scoop batter into rings.
Bake10 minutes.

Topping:

3 Tbsp (45ml) sugar free syrup,

1 Tbsp (15ml) cinnamon swirl whey protein

Pinch of cinnamon (or vanilla)

Macronutrients (per serve):

Protein: 5g

Carbs: 9g

Fat: 1g

Calories: 55

Blueberry Protein Donuts

Serves: 4

Preparation time: 10 minutes

Cooking time: 10 minutes

Ingredients:

⅔ cup (165ml) dry Quaker Old Fashioned Oats

3 large Egg Whites

¼ tsp (1ml) Cinnamon

⅓ cup (85ml) Blueberries

½ tsp (2,5ml) Baking Powder

1 Tbsp (15ml) Bob's Red Mill Almond Meal Flour

½ tsp (2,5ml) Tone's Pure Almond Extract

½ tsp (2,5ml) McCormick Pure Vanilla Extract

½ scoop (20g) Dymatize Nutrition ISO 100 Hydrolyzed 100% Whey Protein Isolate

2 packets Sugar in the Raw or Stevia in The Raw

Method:

Preheat the oven to 350 F (180 C)

Grind the oats into a flour.

Add the rest of the ingredients except for the blueberries and blend again.

Swirl in the blueberries with a spoon.

Spray a donut pan with nonstick spray, and scoop batter into rings.

Bake for 10 minutes. take out and allow to cool.

Topping: (optional)

3 Tbsp (45ml) sugar free maple syrup, with
1 Tbsp (15ml)vanilla whey protein
Pinch of cinnamon

Macronutrients (per donut):

Protein: 7g
Carbs: 7g
Fat: 1.5g

Calories: 71

Chocolate Protein Donuts

Serves: multiple
Preparation time: 10 minutes
Cooking time: 15 minutes

Servings: 4

Ingredients:

1 tsp (5ml) Baking Powder
2 Tbsp (30 ml) Almond Meal Flour
⅓ cup (85ml)Almond Breeze Unsweetened Vanilla Milk
3 Tbsp (45ml) Smith Pure Pumpkin
½ scoop (15g) Pure Protein 100% Whey Protein - Frosty
Chocolate
½ scoop (15g) Muscle Milk Light Vanilla Creme Protein
Powder
4 Tbsp (60ml) Coconut Milk Yogurt - Vanilla

Method:

Preheat the oven to 350 F (180 C)
Batter:
Mix the almond meal, chocolate protein powder,
unsweetened almond milk, chocolate extract, baking
powder, and the pure pumpkin.
Spray a donut pan with nonstick spray, and scoop batter
into rings.
Bake for 15 minutes. take out and allow to cool.
Frosting:
Mix the dairy free yogurt and vanilla protein powder.
Pour over donuts once cooled. Top with chopped nuts or
sprinkles.

Macronutrients (per serve):

Protein: 23g
Carbs: 26g
Fat: 13g

Calories: 294

Protein Packed Parfait

Serves: 1
Preparation time: 10 minutes
Cooking time: None

Ingredients:

1 scoop (30g) Gaspari ISO Fusion Protein Powder
1 Tbsp (15ml) Nescafe Instant Coffee
1 Tbsp (15ml) Cocoa powder
1 cup (250ml) Fage 0% Non-Fat Greek Yogurt
2 Tbsp (30ml) powdered Peanut Putter
⅓ cup (85ml) organic Granola
A few Fresh Blueberries
1 Tbsp (15ml) Dark Chocolate Chips

Method:

Place the granola into to a jar, glass, cup or bowl.
Add ⅓ cup (85ml) yogurt on top of the granola.
Mix ⅓ cup (85ml) yogurt with powdered peanut butter.
Add to the jar.
Mix ⅓ cup (85ml) yogurt with protein powder, coffee, and cocoa powder. Add to the jar.
Top parfait with granola, chocolate chips, and blueberries.

Macronutrients:

Protein: 55 g
Carbs: 34 g
Fat: 9 g

Calories: 435

Coconut-Oat Bars

Serves: 2
Preparation time: 5 Minutes
Cooking time: None

Ingredients:

½ cup (125ml) Oats
½ cup (125ml) liquid Egg Whites
½ scoop (15g) Vanilla Protein
2 Tbsp (30ml) Reduced-Fat unsweetened Coconut Flakes
½ tsp (2.5ml) Coconut Extract
Cinnamon and Stevia to taste
Splash of unsweetened coconut milk

Method:

Preheat oven to 375 F (180 C)
Spray 8x8 pan with non-stick spray.
Blend all ingredients in a blender and pour into pan.
Bake for 15 minutes.
Cut into squares.

Macronutrients (per serve):
Protein: 22 g
Carbs: 21g
Fat: 3 g

Calories: 116

Cinnamon Scroll

Serves: Multiple
Preparation time: 5 Minutes
Cooking time: 15 Minutes

Ingredients:

Cake:
1/2 cup (125ml) liquid Egg Whites
1/2 cup (125ml) MyoFusion Cinnamon Roll Protein
Powder
2 Tbsp (30ml) Oat Flour or instant Buckwheat
1 tsp (5ml) Baking Soda
1 Whole Egg
Frosting:
1/2 cup (125ml) Vanilla Whey
1/2 cup (125ml) Low Fat Greek yogurt
1 tsp (5ml) sugar-free maple syrup

Method:

Cake:
Preheat oven to 390 F (200 C)

Blend all ingredients for cake together.
Pour batter into a large brownie pan. Bake for 10-15
minutes.
When the cake is done, you'll notice it's pretty flat—kind
of like a pancake—this is what we want. Allow to cool.

Frosting:
Combine all ingredients for frosting in a mixing bowl.
After cake is cooled, slice it into three or four strips and

then coat each strip with frosting.

Sprinkle with cinnamon. Be sure to leave some frosting for topping.

Roll each cake strip to create the cinnamon roll.

Macronutrients:

Protein: 44g

Carbs: 11.4g

Fat: 4g

Calories: 290

Strawberry Cheesecake

Servings: 2

Preparation time: 15 Minutes

Cooking time: 45 Minutes

Ingredients:

Crust

¼ cup (62ml) Trader Joe's Just Almond Meal

¼ cup (62ml) shredded Dried Coconut (Shredded, Sweetened)

1 Tbsp (15ml) Coconut Oil

Filling

1 large Egg

1 large Egg White

1 Tbsp (15ml) Fresh Lemon Juice

1 cup (250 ml) 1% Lowfat Cottage Cheese, not packed

2 Tbsp (30ml) Cream Cheese (Fat Free)

1 scoop Body Fortress 100% Premium Vanilla Whey Protein

¾ cup (180ml) Liberte Greek Yogurt 0%

Topping

1 cup, (250ml) pureed Strawberries

2 Tbsp (30ml) Dried Chia Seeds

Method:

Preheat the oven to 190 C (375 F)

Crust:

Coat a pie dish with nonstick spray.

Mix almond meal, shredded coconut and coconut oil together in a mixing bowl.

Place in pie dish and press down to form crust.

Bake for 10 minutes at 190 C (375 F). Remove and let

cool.

Filling:

Mix the egg, egg white, cottage cheese, Greek yogurt, fat free cream cheese, vanilla whey together in a mixing bowl, until smooth.

Add the fresh lemon juice and mix well.

Pour filling into the crust and even it out. Bake for 30-35 minutes at 190 C (375 F).

Take out and let cool.

Toppings:

Mix the strawberry puree and chia seeds together.

Spread over the cheesecake.

Macronutrients (per serving):

Protein: 27g

Carbs: 40g

Fat: 10g

Calories: 365

Smoothies & Shakes

Chocolate Cookie Butter Mass Gain Smoothie

Meal Replacement Shake

Mass Gain Protein Shake (Without Protein Powder)

Iced Green Tea

Hard Gainer Shake

Breakfast Shake

Berry Blast Shake

Orange Creamsickle Protein Shake

Tuna Shake

Banana Bread Shake

Popeye Spinach Shake

Mocha Frappuccino

Pumpkin Protein Smoothie

Avocado Smoothie

Powder-less Protein Shake

Strawberry Cheesecake Protein Smoothie

Chocolate Cookie Butter Mass Gain Smoothie

Serves: 1
Preparation time: 5 Minutes
Cooking time: None

Ingredients:

2 scoops (60g) Chocolate Whey Powder
½ cup (125ml) Ice Water
¼ cup (62ml) Quick Oats
2 Tbsp (30ml) Cookie Butter
1/2 cup (125ml) frozen Greek Yogurt

Method:

Place all the ingredients in blender and blend to desired consistency. Consume immediately.

Macronutrients:

Protein: 52g
Carbs: 80g
Fat: 21g

Calories: 730

Meal Replacement Shake

Serves: 1
Preparation time: 5 Minutes
Cooking time: None

Ingredients:

1 cup (250ml) uncooked Oatmeal
2 scoops (60g)Vanilla protein
¼ tsp (2ml) Cinnamon
2 Tbsp (30ml) Sugar Free Maple Syrup
1 Tbsp (15ml) chopped Almonds
1½ cups (350ml) Water or Low Fat Milk

Method:

Place all the ingredients in blender and blend to desired consistency. Consume immediately.

Macronutrients:

Protein: 68g
Carbs: 33g
Fat: 7g

Calories: 469

Mass Gain Protein Shake (Without Protein Powder)

Serves: 1
Preparation time: 5 Minutes
Cooking time: None

Ingredients:

4 Ice cubes
1 cup (250ml) Water
½ Egg Whites, Liquid
1 Banana, sliced
1 Tbsp (15ml) Peanut Butter
1 tub (130g) Nestlé Greek Yogurt

Method:

Place all the ingredients in blender and blend to desired consistency. Consume immediately.

Macronutrients:

Protein: 25g
Carbs: 55g
Fat: 12g

Calories: 428

Iced Green Tea

Serves: Multiple
Preparation time: 15 Minutes
Chilling time: 3 Hours

Ingredients:

4 cups (1ℓ) Water
2 Green Tea bags
Juice from 1 Lemon
2 Tbsp (30ml) of Honey (optional)
Sprig of Mint
Ice cubes

Method:

Bring the four cups of water to a boil, then pour into a pitcher with the tea bags.
Add the lemon juice, mint leaves, and honey into the tea, and let it steep for 10 minutes.
Remove the teabags and chill.

Add ice cubes and serve cold.

Macronutrients:

Protein: 1g
Carbs: 1g
Fat: 0g

Calories: 8

Hard Gainer Shake

Serves: 2
Preparation time: 10 Minutes
Cooking time: 2 Minutes

Ingredients:

1 cup (250ml) Peanut Butter
½ cup (125ml) Nutella
½ cup (125ml) Oats
2 cups (500ml) 2% Low Fat Milk
1 Banana, sliced
1 tsp (5ml) Cinnamon

Method:

Mix the oats, cinnamon and 1 cup of milk in a microwave proof bowl, and cook for 1minute on high. Remove, stir and cook for another minute.

Scoop the cooked oatmeal mixture into a blender, and blend until smooth.

Add the peanut butter, Nutella, banana and remaining cup of milk, and blend until smooth.

Consume immediately.

Macronutrients (per serve):

Protein: 47g
Carbs: 117g
Fat: 94g

Calories: 1502

Breakfast Shake

Serves: 1
Preparation time: 5 Minutes
Cooking time: None

Ingredients:

2 scoops (60g) Vanilla or Chocolate Protein Powder
1 Banana sliced
¼ cup (62ml) frozen Blueberries
¼ cup (62ml) frozen Black Cherries
¼ cup (62ml) shredded Coconut
⅓ tsp (2ml) Lemon Juice

Method:

Place all the ingredients in blender and blend to desired consistency. Consume immediately.

Macronutrients:

Protein: 65g
Carbs: 30g
Fat: 7g

Calories: 445

Berry Blast Shake

Serves: 2
Preparation time: 5 Minutes
Cooking time: None

Ingredients:

5 Ice cubes
1 cup (250ml) Blueberries
¼ cup (62ml) chopped Cashews
¼ cup (62ml) sliced Almonds
½ cup (125ml) Full-Fat Cottage Cheese
4 scoops (120g) of Vanilla Protein Powder
2 cups (500ml) Milk
¼ tsp (1ml) ground Cinnamon
1 Banana, sliced
1 Tbsp (5ml) Peanut Butter

Method:

Place all the ingredients in blender and blend to desired consistency. Consume immediately.

Macronutrients (per serve):

Protein: 73g
Carbs: 29g
Fat: 18g

Calories: 570

Orange Creamsickle Protein Shake

Serves: 1
Preparation time: 5 Minutes
Cooking time: None

Ingredients:

1 cup (250ml) Ice
1 cup (250ml) Orange Juice
1 scoop (30g) Vanilla Whey
1 tsp (5ml) Vanilla Extract
2 Tbsp (30ml) Non Fat Plain Greek Yogurt

Method:

Place all the ingredients in blender and blend to desired consistency. Consume immediately.

Macronutrients:

Protein: 33g
Carbs: 25g
Fat: 3g

Calories: 259

Tuna Shake

Serves: 1
Preparation time: 5 Minutes
Cooking time: None

Ingredients:

2 6oz cans (340g) Tuna, drained
2 cups (500ml) Water
4 Large Ice cubes

Method:

Place all the ingredients in blender and blend to desired
consistency. Consume immediately.

Macronutrients:

Protein: 80g
Carbs: 4g
Fat: 0g

Calories: 336

Banana Bread Shake

Serves: 1
Preparation time: 5 Minutes
Cooking time: None

Ingredients:

2 scoops (60g) Vanilla Whey Protein
1 Banana, peeled and sliced
½ cup (125ml) Quaker Oatmeal (cooked in water)
½ cup (125ml) Bran Flakes
1½ cup (350ml) Water
30g of Dextrose (Only if consumed post-workout)

Method:

Place all the ingredients in blender and blend to desired consistency. Consume immediately.

Macronutrients:

Protein: 56g
Carbs: 64g (34 without Dextrose)
Fat: 2g

Calories: 498

Popeye Spinach Shake

Serves: 1
Preparation time: 5 Minutes
Cooking time: None

Ingredients:

1½ cups (375ml) Water
1 - 1½ cups (375ml) leafy Spinach
2 Tbsp (30ml) Almond Butter
2 scoops (30g) Whey Protein
4 cubes Ice

Method:

Place all the ingredients in blender and blend to desired consistency. Consume immediately.

Macronutrients:

Protein: 56g
Carbs: 10g
Fat: 19g

Calories: 424

Mocha Frappuccino

Serves: 1
Preparation time: 5 Minutes
Cooking time: None

Ingredients:

1 tsp (5ml) instant coffee granules of your choice
1 scoop (30g) Chocolate Whey Protein
1½ cup (375 ml) Crushed Ice = 10-15 ice cubes
1 cup (250ml)Skimmed Milk
2-3 packs Splenda

Method:

Place all the ingredients in blender and blend to desired consistency. Consume immediately.

Macronutrients:

Protein: 43g
Carbs: 8g
Fat: 2g

Calories: 222

Pumpkin Protein Smoothie

Serves: 1
Preparation time: 5 Minutes
Cooking time: None

Ingredients:

1½ scoops (45g) Double Chocolate Whey
½ Can Libby's Canned Pumpkin Puree
1 Packet Splenda or Honey
½ cup (125ml) Water
6 Ice cubes

Method:

Place all the ingredients in blender and blend to desired consistency. Consume immediately.

Macronutrients:

Protein: 40g
Carbs: 22.5g
Fat: 1.5g

Calories: 260

Avocado Smoothie

Serves: 2
Preparation time: 5 Minutes
Cooking time: None

Ingredients:

1 Medium Avocado, peeled and diced
1 cup (250ml) Almond Milk
1 tsp (5ml) Honey
¼ - ½ tsp (2-2,5ml) Vanilla Extract

Method:

Place all the ingredients in blender and blend to desired consistency. Consume immediately.

Macronutrients:

Protein: 3g
Carbs: 17g
Fat: 13g

Calories: 180

Serves: 1
Preparation time: 10 Minutes
Cooking time: None

Ingredients:

¾ Cup (190ml) Sugar Free Vanilla Coconut Milk (or Milk Substitute)
½ tsp (2,5ml)Vanilla Extract
½ tsp (2,5ml) Ground Cinnamon
1 Tub (5.3 Ounces/150g) Vanilla Fat Free Greek Yogurt
¼ cup (62ml) Fat Free Cottage Cheese
1 Tbsp (15ml) Peanut Butter
9 Tbsp (135ml) Liquid Egg Whites
1 Tbsp (15ml) Instant Sugar Free Fat Free Vanilla Pudding
Ice (Optional)

Method:

Place all the ingredients in blender and blend to desired consistency. Consume immediately.

Macronutrients:

Protein: 31g
Carbs: 27g
Fat: 7g

Calories: 295

Strawberry Cheesecake Protein Smoothie

Serves: 1
Preparation time: 10 Minutes
Cooking time: None

Ingredients:

1 cup (250ml) Sugar Free Vanilla Coconut Milk (or milk substitute)
3 Tbsp (45ml) Liquid Egg Whites
1 Tbsp (15ml) Instant Sugar Free Fat Free Cheesecake Jello
1 cup (250ml) Halved Strawberries
1/2 cup (125ml) Fat Free Cottage Cheese
1½ scoops (45g) Strawberry or Vanilla Protein Powder
1/2 tsp (5ml)Vanilla Extract
1 cup (250ml) Ice

Method:

Place all the ingredients in blender and blend to desired consistency. Consume immediately.

Macronutrients:

Protein: 59g
Carbs: 30g
Fat: 6g

Calories: 410

Sides

Low Calorie Chocolate Sauce

Athlete Trail Mix

High Protein Ranch Sauce

Tuna Dip

Shrimp Ceviche

Shrimp Sliders

Turkey-Wrapped Asparagus

Cupcake Frosting

Scallop Cerviche

Cinnamon Sweet Potato Fries

Clean Protein Nutella Spread

Low Calorie Chocolate Sauce

Serves: multiple
Preparation time: 5 Minutes
Cooking time: None

Ingredients:

5g Cocoa or powdered Hot Chocolate of your choice
2 tsp (10ml) Canderel/Splenda/Sweetener of choice
½ tsp (2,5ml)Vanilla Extract.
½ Tsp (2,5ml) Xanthan Gum.
Small amount of boiling Water

Method:

Combine the cocoa, sweetner and Xanthan gum in a cup.
Add the vanilla extract and smix well.
Add increments of boiling water to the mixture, until the
desired consistency is obtained – should you add too
much water, add a small amount of Xanthan gum.
Leave to cool/set, or use immediately.

Macronutrients:

Protein: 1g
Carbs: 0g
Fat: 4g

Calories: 28

Athlete Trail Mix

Serves: multiple
Preparation time: 5 Minutes
Cooking time: None

Ingredients:

½ cup (125ml) Dairy free, gluten free chocolate chips
½ cup (125ml) Pumpkin seeds
½ cup (125ml) Sunflower seeds
½ cup (125ml) Banana Chips
½ cup (125ml) Dried Cranberries
½ cup (125ml) Shredded Coconut

(Or whichever dried fruits/nuts you prefer!)

Method:

Place all ingredients in a mixing bowl and mix well.

Seal in an airtight container, or pack into small snack-sized ziplock bags.

Snack on as desired.

Macronutrients:

Macronutrient breakdown and total number of calories is hard to determine with trail mix, however I recommend experimenting with your favourite seeds and nuts, and obtaining a baseline from these calories.

High Protein Ranch Sauce

Servings: Multiple
Preparation time: 10 Minutes
Cooking time: None

Ingredients:

6oz (170g) Fat Free Plain Greek Yogurt
9 Tbsp (135ml) Fat Free Sour Cream
¼ tsp (2ml) Dill, chopped
1 tsp (5ml) Parsley, chopped
3/4 tsp (3ml) Salt
½ tsp (2,5ml) Onion Powder
¼ tsp (2ml) Garlic Powder
¼ tsp(2ml) Black Pepper
Water (until desired consistency)
1/2 Scoop (15g) Natural Flavored Protein Powder
(optional)

Method:

Place all of the ingredients in a mixing bowl and mix well.
Add in water until the sauce has obtained your desired
consistency (the less water you use the creamier it'll be).
Add a natural flavored protein powder if you want more
protein.

Macronutrients:

Protein: 34g
Carbs: 23g
Fat: 0g

Calories: 228

Tuna Dip

Servings: Multiple
Preparation time: 5 Minutes
Cooking time: None

Ingredients:

1 Can (5 Ounces/142g) Tuna
⅓ Packet Ranch Dip
2 Tbsp (30ml) Flax Seed
1 Container (6 Ounces/170g) Plain Fat Free Greek Yogurt

Method:

Drain your can of Tuna.
Place in a mixing bowl, add the ranch dip, flax seed and yogurt and mix well.
Serve immediately with snacks.

Macronutrients:

Protein: 47g
Carbs:16g
Fat: 5g

Calories: 297

Shrimp Ceviche

Servings: 4
Preparation time: 5 Minutes
Cooking time: None

Ingredients:

½ lb (225g) Large shrimp, cooked, peeled and chopped
½ cup (125ml) Cherry Tomatoes, sliced
¼ Red Onion, sliced
¼ cup (62ml) Cilantro, chopped
½ Avocado, chopped
Juice of 1 Lime
Salt and Pepper, to taste

Method:

Add ingredients to a medium bowl.
Toss and refrigerate before serving.

Macronutrients (per serving):

Protein: 12.5g
Carbs: 5.5g
Fat: 4.4g

Calories: 111

Servings: 3
Preparation time: 5 Minutes
Cooking time: None

Ingredients:

6 oz (170g) raw Shrimp, de-veined and peeled
3 Ozery Bakery multigrain slider buns
½ cup (125ml) Bell Pepper, diced
1 Roma Tomato, sliced
Lettuce leaves
½ Tbsp (7,5ml) Kelapo Coconut oil or use the spray

Seasonings:
Onion powder,
Garlic powder,
Pepper,
Cumin

Method:

Wash and remove all tails and peel the raw shrimp and
Dry the shrimp with a paper towel.
Add the shrimp to a blender and pulse blend until a
chunky, thick sticky paste is achieved.
Remove the shrimp from the food processor and season
with your choice of seasonings.

Mix using your hands, and form three equal sized patties.

Heat a skillet on medium heat and add the Kelapo
coconut oil. (If you are placing the shrimp on the grill, be
sure to grease the rack.)

Place the shrimp sliders on the skillet and cook until the shrimp patties turn pink.

Assemble the sliders using a small leaf of lettuce and a slice of Roma tomato.

Serve immediately.

Macronutrients (per serving):

Serving size 1 slider
Protein: 14g
Carbs:13g
Fat: 2g

Calories: 135

Turkey-Wrapped Asparagus

Servings: 12
Preparation time: 10 Minutes
Cooking time: 10 Minutes

Ingredients:

A bundle of thick spears of Asparagus (roughly 12)
24oz (600g) Turkey Lunchmeat, sliced thinly
Kelapo Coconut Oil

Seasonings (optional):
Bragg's Liquid Aminos,
Garlic powder,
Onion powder

Instructions:

Preheat oven to 450 F (220 C)
Spray a baking sheet with a nonstick spray

Chop bottom stems off asparagus.
Wrap each asparagus with 2 oz of sliced turkey lunch meat.
Heat a skillet over a medium-high flame and spray with Kelapo coconut oil.
Place the wrapped asparagus in the skillet with the turkey flap end down.
Sear the wrapped asparagus.
While cooking, add seasoning.

Once all sides of the turkey are seared, remove from the skillet.

Place the wrapped asparagus in the oven on a baking sheet and bake in the oven for 4-5 minutes.

Serve warm.

Macronutrients (per serving):

Serving size: One asparagus wrap

Protein:12g
Carbs: 2g
Fat: 1g

Calories: 66

Cupcake Frosting

Servings: Multiple
Preparation time: 5 Minutes
Cooking time: None

Ingredients:

2 scoops casein protein powder (½ - ¾ cup, depending on desired thickness)
1 cup (250ml) Greek yogurt
5 Tbsp (75ml) Milk

Method:

Place the protein powder and yogurt together in a bowl, and mix.

Stir in one tablespoon of milk at a time, until the mixture acquires a frosting like texture. It should be creamy and not overly runny. Feel free to add more casein if you want thicker frosting, or more yogurt if you want it creamier.

When casein mixture is ready, use it to frost your cooled muffins. You can either use a knife to spread it, or put the frosting in a Ziploc bag, cut off a corner, and use it as a frosting bag.

Macronutrients:

Protein: 75g
Carbs: 5g
Fat: 5g

Calories:

Scallop Cerviche

Serves: 3
Preparation time: Overnight
Cooking time: None

Ingredients:

1 lb (450g) Bay Scallops (these are small scallops, roughly
the size of a marble)
Juice of 6 Limes (enough to cover the scallops – you can
use lemons if you prefer)
½ large Red Onion chopped
1 medium sized Tomato
1 stalk of Celery
2 Tbsp (30ml) of Capers
2 Tbsp (30ml) Olive Oil
Pinch of Sea Salt
1 tsp (5ml) ground Black Pepper (or to taste)

Method:

Place the scallops into a shallow bowl and squeeze the
juice from the limes over the scallops.
Cover and refrigerate for 4-8 hours (overnight).

Remove from the refrigerator, and drain off most of the
limejuice.

Dice the onion, tomato, and celery, and add it to the
scallops along with the capers, salt, olive oil and pepper.

Refrigerate for another hour and serve cold.

Macronutrients (per serving):

Protein: 26g
Carbs: 7g
Fat: 10g

Calories: 241

Cinnamon Sweet Potato Fries

Serves: 1
Preparation time: 10 Minutes
Cooking time: 20 Minutes

Ingredients:

½ tbsp (7.5ml) Cinnamon
250 g Sweet Potato
¼ cup (62ml) Extra Virgin Olive Oil
½ scoop (15g) Cellucor Cor-Performance Whey

Method:

Preheat your oven to 425 F (200 C)
Wash and dry your sweet potato, peel if preferred.
Coat a baking tray with nonstick cooking spray.

Slice into fries – ensure that they are all about the same width.
Place the olive oil and Cinnamon Swirl protein in a mixing bowl, and mix well.
Coat all your fries and place on a baking sheet, ensure that the fries are evenly spaced.
Sprinkle with cinnamon.
Bake for 15-20 minutes at depending on how thick your fries are.

Check every 5 minutes or so. You may want to flip them ½ or ¾ the way through.

Serve hot

Macronutrients (per serving):

Protein: 8g
Carbs: 27g
Fat: 27g

Calories: 383

Clean Protein Nutella Spread

Serves: Multiple
Preparation time: 10 Minutes
Cooking time: 10 Minutes

Ingredients:

2 cups (500ml) Raw Hazelnuts
1½ tbsp (22.5ml) pure Vanilla Extract
¼ cup (63ml) Cacao Powder
¼ cup (63ml) Rice Malt Syrup (or other sweetener)
½ cup (125ml) of unsweetened Almond Milk

Method:

Preheat your oven to **Preheat oven to 200 F (1200 C)**
Place the hazelnuts on a baking sheet and roast for 10 minutes.
Remove from the oven and allow to cool.
Using a paper towel, rub the hazelnuts together to remove their darkened skin.
Blend the nuts in a food processor until smooth and buttery.
Add the Cacao powder, sweetener, vanilla extract and almond milk,
Blend well until smooth.
Store in an airtight jar or container in a cool place until ready to use.

Macronutrients:

Protein: 38g
Carbs: 50g
Fat: 90g

Calories: 1162

Conclusion

I hope these recipes will serve you well on the way to achieving your health and fitness goals. Once you've got these recipes mastered don't be shy to add extra ingredients and flavours, as well as alter the amount of protein/carbohydrates based ingredients in each dish to better suit your calorie and macronutrient goals.

I'd love to hear your success stories with these recipes, and your overall thoughts on the Flexible Dieting Cook Book – feel free to submit a review via Amazon.

Happy cooking!

Scott James

CPSIA information can be obtained at www.ICGtesting.com
Printed in the USA
BVOW06s0526031215

429167BV00072B/365/P